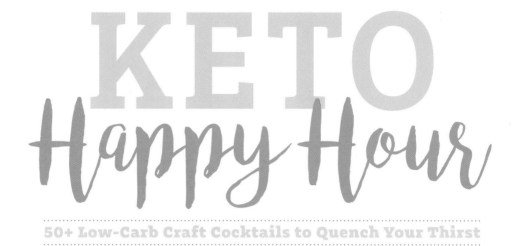

KETO
Happy Hour

50+ Low-Carb Craft Cocktails to Quench Your Thirst

Kyndra D. Holley

D0565803

Victory Belt Publishing Inc.
Las Vegas

Front and back cover photography by Hayley Mason and Bill Staley
Cheesy Nachos photo on page 183 by Kelly Bejelly
Interior design by Yordan Terziev and Boryana Yordanova

Printed in Canada

TC 0318

CONTENTS

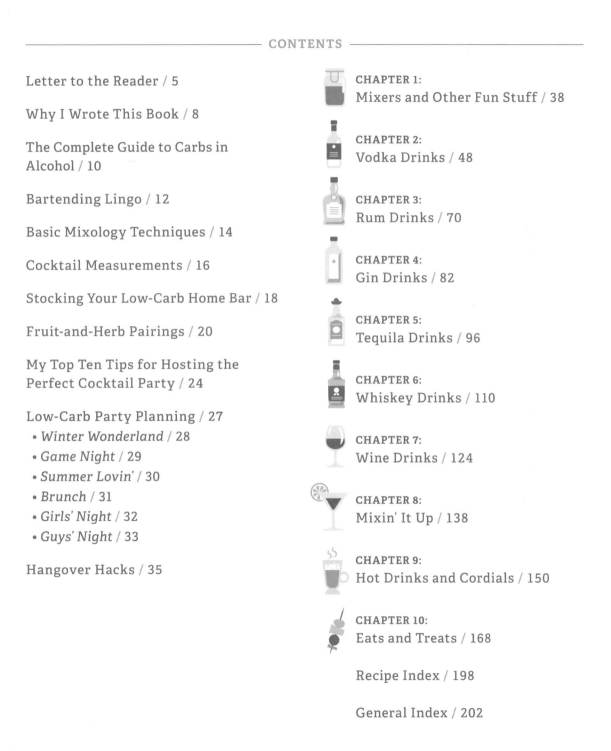

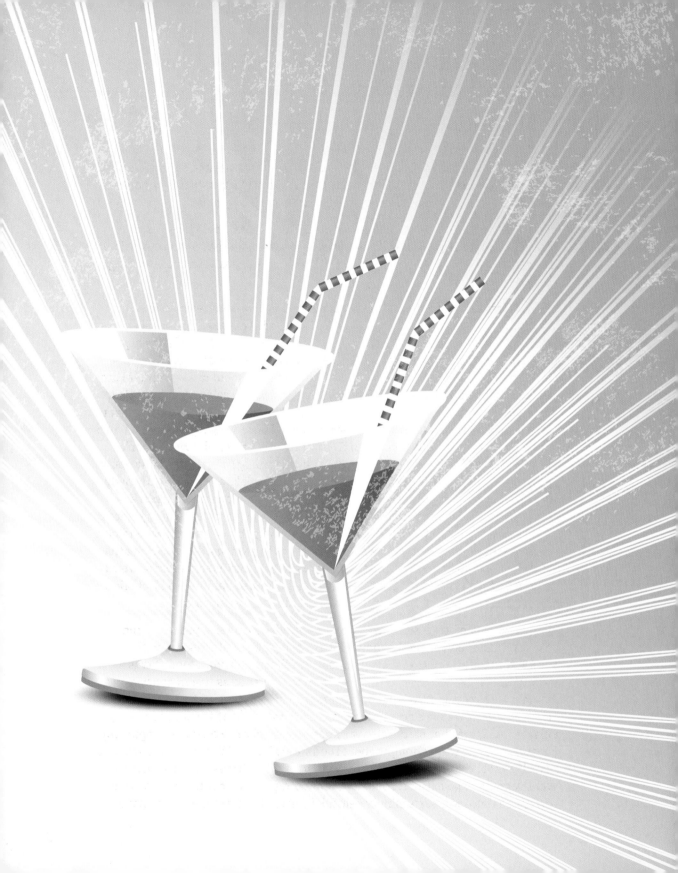

Letter to the Reader

Hello, all my libation-loving friends! It's time to raise a glass and say cheers to *Keto Happy Hour*! Cheers! *Salud! Saúde! Cincin! Santé! Proost!* In my world, as long as you are happy and healthy, then it is always happy hour.

You might be asking yourself, "A low-carb cocktail book? Could it be possible? Has Kyndra finally gone mad?" Well, I am here to tell you that, yes, it is possible. You can, in fact, have most of your favorite cocktails in healthier low-carb, sugar-free versions.

When I first set out to live a low-carb lifestyle, I immediately learned that if I was going to have any success at all, I had to rethink the way I did just about everything where food and beverages were concerned. I had to redefine my emotional relationship with food. You see, food used to control me. I lived in a self-perpetuated world where food was either a punishment or a reward. If I ate perfectly for two weeks and got my workouts in, I would celebrate with a big ol' food-and-drink bingefest that typically included a lot of excess carbs and sugar. What I was doing to myself was the equivalent of rewarding my dogs with treats for being good on a walk or going to the bathroom outside. Silly, right? Don't reward yourself with food—you are not a dog. The only thing I was really doing was undoing all the hard work of the previous two weeks and making my body work even harder to get back on track. I was feeding it a bunch of processed foods, carbs, and sugar and then asking it not to crave them the next day—not a genius move. Some of you might not like this analogy, but when you are addicted to carbs and sugar and you have successfully gone through a detox period after which you are no longer craving them, eating them again as some sort of weird reward that you've told yourself you deserve is a lot like handing an alcoholic a beer and asking him to drink only that one and not crave any more.

If you own any of my other books or have ever visited my site, peaceloveand-lowcarb.com, then you likely know a lot about my personal struggles with weight and my attempts to fix my unhealthy relationship with food. It was a very long road to recovery before I was able to view food as fuel to nourish and support a healthy and thriving body. I am the type of person who, as soon as I tell myself or someone else tells me that I can't have something, it becomes my sole desire. Given that bit of self-awareness, I learned early on that changing my lifestyle and the way I thought about food would be no different. I had to remind myself that there was not going to be any great pizza famine and that potatoes weren't going to go extinct. Somehow, reminding myself that those foods would always be there was surprisingly helpful. I started telling myself, "I can have that tomorrow." Then, the next day, I would say the same thing. Tomorrow would come and I would say again, "Tomorrow. I can have that tomorrow." After enough tomorrows had passed, I no longer craved those high-carb foods that I'd so desperately wanted. Granting myself permission to eat it tomorrow instead of telling myself that I could never have it again was oddly comforting. In my heart, I knew I wasn't going to eat a high-carb delivery pizza or a bag of potato chips tomorrow, but somehow, giving myself grace and permission helped me find the fortitude to push forward. Eventually, I no longer needed permission to eat those foods because I no longer wanted them. Plus, I discovered about a million different ways to make low-carb pizza that scratched the pizza itch just fine.

In fact, my blog was born because I set out on a mission to re-create my favorite foods in healthier low-carb versions instead of just taking them all off the table completely. I guess you could say that my specialty is low-carb comfort food. I learned how to stop viewing food as a reward, and in return, I was able to put all my favorite foods back on the table in a manner that did not leave me feeling deprived or like I needed to apologize to my body the next day.

So what does all this have to do with happy hour or alcoholic beverages, you might ask? Well, long after I had fixed my relationship with food, I was still indulging in cocktails almost as if they were a free food—as if a magic fairy had come down from the sky and sprinkled fairy dust on my drink, removing all of its carbs and sugar. I was eating well, working out, and then undoing all my hard work at happy hour. I knew I needed to clean up my happy hour routine as well if I wanted to continue achieving my health and weight-loss goals. At the same time, I was smart enough to apply the same principles I had with food to drinks. I knew that if I told myself I was never going to go out for drinks with friends again, it would become a fixation. I'm just so darn defiant in that way—a rebel for the sake of rebelling. Sure, I could have gone out with friends and had a club soda, but why lead myself into a situation of extreme temptation when I could simply change up my routine and find a happy medium? I realized that I didn't have to give up my social life to achieve my weight-loss goals. I just needed to get creative with what I was eating and drinking.

I bartended for a lot of the years I spent working in restaurants. I loved it. It was such a rush being behind the bar on a Friday night, making drink after drink as fast as my hands could possibly move. With that came a lot of drink sampling, and then a lot of actual drinking after my shift ended. In restaurant work, and in a lot of other fields that involve shift work, going out to eat and drink after work becomes your whole social life. We live in a society where, in most social circles, social events are synonymous with cocktails: weddings, sporting events, New Year's Eve, tropical vacations . . . I could go on and on. When was the last time you were at any type of social gathering that did not include alcohol of some sort?

Sure, there are plenty of dry events, too, but chances are that if you are reading this book, those probably aren't the kinds of events you are attending.

Keto Happy Hour will help you stay true to your keto lifestyle in all types of social settings. Whether you are learning how to choose the lowest-carb option during a night out or you are planning to host a low-carb gathering that won't leave you feeling deprived, this book will help you incorporate the occasional cocktail into your low-carb lifestyle. Can we all raise a glass to that? CHEERS!!

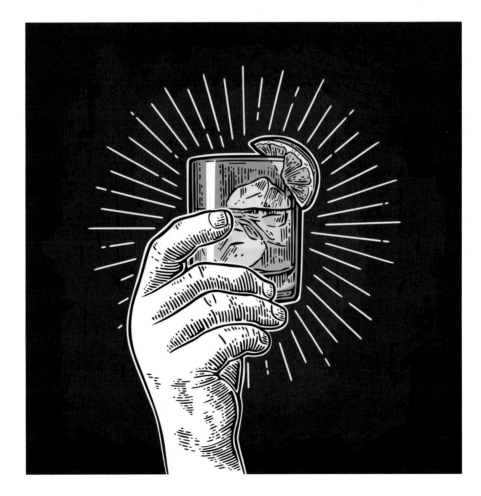

Why I Wrote This Book

When you're switching to a new lifestyle and way of eating, it can be hard to find your social groove again. You start to realize how many of your interactions with friends and family are centered around food and drinks. You become abundantly aware of all the food around you that you can no longer eat. It almost makes you more food-centric than you were before. You start noticing that those cocktails that you used to throw back with reckless abandon are inching you further away from your health and weight-loss goals. As you start to learn new food habits, form a healthier relationship with food, and focus more on what you are putting in your body, social gatherings can be stressful and downright anxiety-inducing. Constantly turning down food as it passes by you, questioning every single ingredient in the mixed drinks, and explaining your new lifestyle choices over and over again can take a lot of the joy out of social events that were once happy and carefree occasions.

In addition, including alcohol in a low-carb, ketogenic way of life may seem like an indulgent no-no. Sorting through the vast number of studies, personal testimonials, and scientific information advocating for and against alcohol can be tricky—it can easily land you in a state of analysis paralysis. Ultimately, what works for one body may not work for another. But I know many people who can enjoy the occasional low-carb cocktail and still reach their health and weight-loss goals, myself included. As with most things, I believe moderation is the key. Just as you can't reach your goals by eating ten slices of low-carb pizza every day, you aren't going to reach your goals by imbibing ten cocktails every day.

Well, it's time to put the "happy" back in happy hour! My main goal in writing this book is to give you as many tools as possible to help you achieve your health and weight-loss goals while maintaining the kind of social life you are accustomed to. I have learned time and time again that while success does require a substantial amount of compromise, it doesn't have to come at the cost of an active social calendar.

I wrote this book for everyone looking to find ease and balance between their active social calendar and their healthy low-carb lifestyle. If you are tired of testing your willpower and explaining your lifestyle choices, it might be time to host your own get-together, and that's what *Keto Happy Hour* is all about. Hosting your own social gatherings puts *you* in charge of the menu so that you can experience food and drink freedom while enjoying yourself in a social setting. Doesn't that sound amazing? With the delicious low-carb food and drink recipes in this book and the Low-Carb Party Planning menus on pages 27 to 33, I've got you covered. Now you can have fun with friends and enjoy delicious low-carb food and drinks at the same time.

The introductory sections of this book (pages 10 to 37) will give you the basics on carbs in alcohol and teach you how to unleash your inner bartender. From basic bartending lingo to mixology techniques, you'll learn everything you need to know to be entertaining with grace and ease in no time flat. I'll explain how to set up the perfect low-carb home bar, right down to the barware and the garnishes. And should you find yourself having so much fun that the night gets away from you, I've even thrown in some tried-and-true hangover hacks. Hey, it happens to the best of us!

Now it's time to think of a theme and host your heart out. Cheers to happy hour!

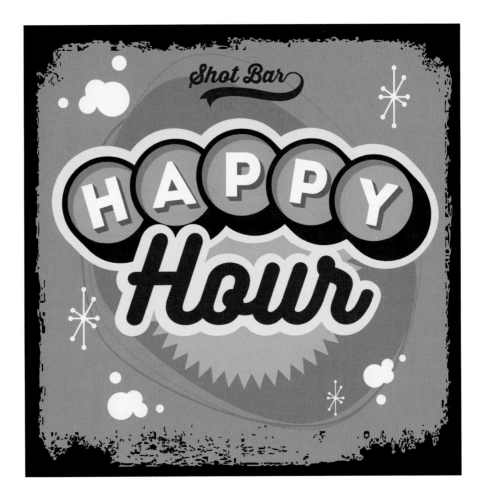

The Complete Guide to Carbs in Alcohol

	Carbs in 5 Fluid Ounces
RED WINE	
Pinot Noir	3.5 g
Merlot	3.7 g
Cabernet Sauvignon	3.8 g
Syrah	3.8 g
Zinfandel	3.8 g
WHITE WINE AND ROSÉ	
Sparkling white	1.5 g
Brut champagne	2.5 g
Sauvignon Blanc	2.8 g
Pinot Grigio	3 g
Chardonnay	3.1 g
SWEET WHITE WINE	
White Zinfandel	5 g
Riesling	5.7 g
Moscato	8 g

WINE

Wine is a great option whether you're entertaining at home or dining out. As long as you stick to dry or semisweet red, white, and sparkling wines, you can rest assured that in most cases a glass of wine will come in at less than 5 grams of carbs, which makes it a safe and easy go-to. It's also a great choice because you always know exactly what you are getting; when ordering a mixed drink, you run the risk of accidentally getting poured a high-carb alcohol or mixer.

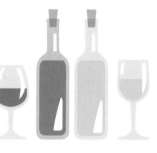

BEER	Carbs in 12 Fluid Ounces
Bud Select 55	1.9 g
Miller 64	2.4 g
Michelob Ultra	2.6 g
Bud Select	3.1 g
Busch Lite	3.2 g
Miller Light	3.2 g
Michelob Ultra Amber	3.7 g
Amstel Light	5 g
Coors Light	5 g
Corona Light	5 g
Bud Light	6.6 g
Heineken Light	6.8 g

BEER

There are thousands of different beers on the market—imported and domestic, craft and microbrew. While many people following a strict low-carb, keto diet omit gluten altogether, for those who do enjoy the occasional beer, I feel it is important to provide a list of the lowest-carb beers on the market. Most of the beers on this list are widely available and should be easy to find at your local grocery store. However, please be advised that none of these beers are gluten-free. If you are looking for a good gluten-free beer option, check out brands like Omission that are crafted to remove gluten. If you have a higher carb allowance or are at a maintenance weight, hard cider is also a delicious option.

LIQUOR

LIQUOR (UNFLAVORED)	Carbs in 1½ Fluid Ounces
Vodka	0
Gin	0
White rum	0
Dark rum	0
Tequila	0
Spiced rum	0.5 g
Whiskey/Bourbon	0 to 3 g*
Brandy	0 to 3 g*

varies by brand

Contrary to popular belief, not all liquors are low-carb and gluten-free. In fact, many are very high in carbs and contain added sugars. It is important to look at each brand individually for product and nutritional information.

However, the table at left is a basic guideline for different kinds of liquor. The best rule to follow when crafting a low-carb cocktail is to stick to plain, unsweetened, unflavored clear liquors, like vodka, gin, and white rum. Tequila and whiskey are also safe bets.

SPIKED SELTZER WATER

BRAND	Carbs in 12 Fluid Ounces
Truly Spiked and Sparkling	2 g
White Claw	4 g
Spiked Seltzer	5 g

The low-carb beverage space is growing rapidly as more people catch on to the health benefits of an overall reduction in carbohydrates, not only in food but in drinks as well. A whole new category is emerging in the form of spiked seltzer waters. Light, with a hint of fruit flavoring, these are a great option for those who aren't fans of strong alcoholic drinks, beer, or wine.

MIXERS AND FLAVOR ENHANCERS

Angostura bitters

Essential oils

Flavored stevia drops

Fresh berries

Fresh citrus fruits

Fresh herbs

Ginger Syrup (page 42)

Kombucha

Low-Carb Simple Syrup (page 40)

Low-Carb Sweet-and-Sour Mix (page 46)

Naturally flavored sparkling water

Naturally flavored sugar-free sodas, such as Zevia

Plain sparkling water, like club soda

Pure extracts

Unsweetened or light cranberry juice

Now that you know which types of alcohol are the safest low-carb options, it's time to decide what to mix them with. Many of the traditional mixers offered in restaurants and bars are loaded with carbs and sugar. The list of low-carb mixers and flavor enhancers at left should have you well on your way to making the wisest choices possible, whether you are dining out or entertaining at home.

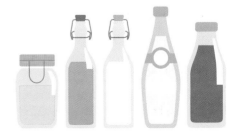

Bartending Lingo

Learning these basic bar terms will have you well on your way to slinging drinks and tossing cocktail shakers and glasses through the air like Tom Cruise in Cocktail. I may be dating myself a bit with that reference, but, hey, some movies are just classics. And so are some cocktails!

This isn't a complete glossary of terms for bartending in general, but rather some of the terms that you will see used throughout this book. With just a little bit of know-how and a desire for fun, you will soon be hosting the hottest low-carb cocktail parties in town.

BACK
A small glass of something (like water, soda, or juice) that accompanies a drink or shot.

CHASER
A neutral-flavored drink, usually nonalcoholic, consumed immediately after a straight shot of liquor to help clear the palate.

COBBLER
A mixed drink that typically consists of a liquor, sugar (or low-carb natural sweetener in this book), and fresh fruit.

COCKTAIL SHAKER
A device into which you pour ingredients and then shake to mix and/or chill a beverage, typically alcoholic. Most cocktail shakers come with a lid and a built-in strainer.

DASH
A few drops or a very small amount of an ingredient.

DIRTY
What makes a drink "dirty" is the addition of some of the juice from its garnish. This is most commonly associated with olive juice in a classic dirty martini, but cocktail onion brine or even pickle juice can be added.

FIZZ
A carbonated cocktail, typically containing club soda.

GARNISH
A decorative, edible ornament that accompanies a mixed drink.

JIGGER A two-sided bar tool used to measure alcohol. Each side holds a different measurement of liquid. Standard double jiggers come in two sizes: ½ ounce on one side and 1 ounce on the other, or ¾ ounce on one side and 1½ ounces on the other. If you ever see "jigger" as a measurement in a cocktail recipe, it is assumed to equal 1½ ounces.

MIXER Nonalcoholic ingredients added to a mixed drink or cocktail.

NEAT A single, unmixed liquor, served at room temperature, without ice and without any sort of mixer.

NIGHTCAP Wine or liquor served right before bedtime.

ON THE ROCKS Poured over ice.

SHOT A straight shot of a single liquor taken neat. Most commonly a 1½- to 2-ounce pour.

TWIST A piece of citrus zest that's twisted into a spiral and used as a cocktail garnish.

UP A drink served chilled but without ice.

VIRGIN DRINK / MOCKTAIL A drink typically made with alcohol that is served with all the same ingredients, minus the alcohol.

WEDGE Fruit cut into a wedge shape for use as a garnish or in cocktail preparation.

WHEEL Fruit sliced into a wheel shape and placed on the rim of a glass as a garnish. Sometimes wheels are cut in half to make to half-moons.

Basic Mixology Techniques

I'm sure you've heard the famous Bond one-liner "Martini, shaken, not stirred." If you are a die-hard fan of the 007 franchise, you probably read that in the voice of Sean Connery. Here is a little-known fact: in the book, it is actually written as "Martini, stirred, not shaken," which makes a lot more sense given that, by the time of Bond, bartenders might just as easily have shaken a martini as stirred it. But what does it all mean? What is the difference between a stirred drink and a shaken one? Is stirring a drink the same as stirring a pot of soup on the stove? Why do you shake a drink? Is floating something you do down a river?

By learning just a few basic mixology techniques, you will be well on your way to making hundreds of different drinks like a pro. Next time someone asks you to muddle some fresh citrus fruit into their cocktail, you will know exactly what they are talking about. Better yet, you can whip out your bar tools and wow them with your master bartending skills before they even ask.

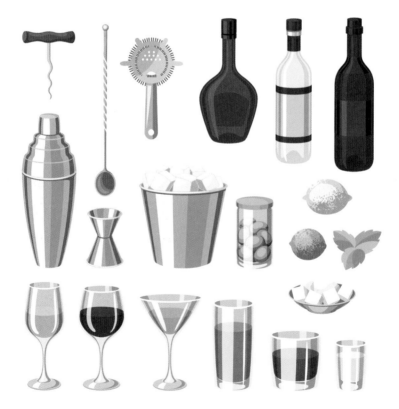

BLEND—Used when referring to blended drinks, also called frozen drinks. This term simply means to mix ingredients and ice in an electric blender.

CHILL—Most often used in reference to martinis. Drinks that are served up, such as martinis, are served in a chilled glass. To chill the glass while you are preparing the drink, fill it with ice and top it off with water. Pour out the ice water before straining the drink into the chilled glass.

FLOAT—When one alcohol or mixer sits on top of another alcohol or mixer, almost as if suspended. Floating can be accomplished by pouring the alcohol very carefully down the side of the glass or by slowly pouring it over the top of an inverted spoon, allowing the alcohol to trickle off the spoon into the drink.

LAYER—Layering a shot or drink is achieved in the same fashion as floating. The heavier alcohol is poured first, and then the lighter alcohol is carefully poured down the side of the glass or over an inverted spoon so that it rests on top of the heavier alcohol.

MUDDLE—To extract flavor and essential oils from ingredients such as fruits and fresh herbs by crushing them with a bar tool called a muddler. A muddler resembles a small baseball bat and is used to repeatedly apply a crushing pressure to ingredients until they have released their oils and juices.

SHAKE—To fill a cocktail shaker with ice, add the ingredients, and then cap and shake to chill the drink and combine the ingredients. Drinks made with juice, cream, egg whites, or "dirty" components, such as olive or pickle brine, are always shaken.

STIR—When a cocktail is ordered "stirred," the drink is made in the same way as a shaken drink, but instead of shaking, a bar spoon is used to stir the drink until it's well chilled, about 20 seconds. Mixed drinks that are built in the serving glass, such as a Vodka Soda (page 53), are often given a stir with a bar spoon to combine the drink components.

STRAIN—To pour out the liquid from a cocktail shaker into a glass while removing the ice and any other solid ingredients.

Cocktail Measurements

As explained in the "Bartending Lingo" section on pages 12 and 13, the jigger is the standard bar tool used for measuring alcohol (and sometimes other liquid ingredients) for a cocktail. While a jigger is ideal, it is not absolutely necessary. You can easily get by with a good set of measuring spoons. Measuring spoons come in especially handy when a recipe calls for an amount not measured on a standard jigger. Standard jiggers come in two sizes, with either ½- and 1-ounce measurements or ¾- and 1½-ounce measurements. But what if you want to pour 1¼ ounces? This conversion chart can help you out with that task. And in case you were wondering, 1¼ ounces would be 2 tablespoons plus 1½ teaspoons.

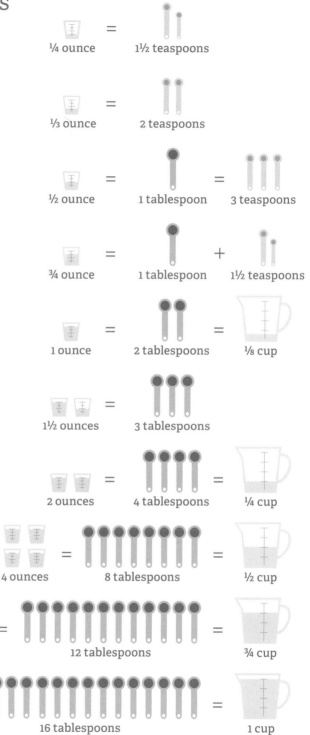

¼ ounce = 1½ teaspoons

⅓ ounce = 2 teaspoons

½ ounce = 1 tablespoon = 3 teaspoons

¾ ounce = 1 tablespoon + 1½ teaspoons

1 ounce = 2 tablespoons = ⅛ cup

1½ ounces = 3 tablespoons

2 ounces = 4 tablespoons = ¼ cup

4 ounces = 8 tablespoons = ½ cup

6 ounces = 12 tablespoons = ¾ cup

8 ounces = 16 tablespoons = 1 cup

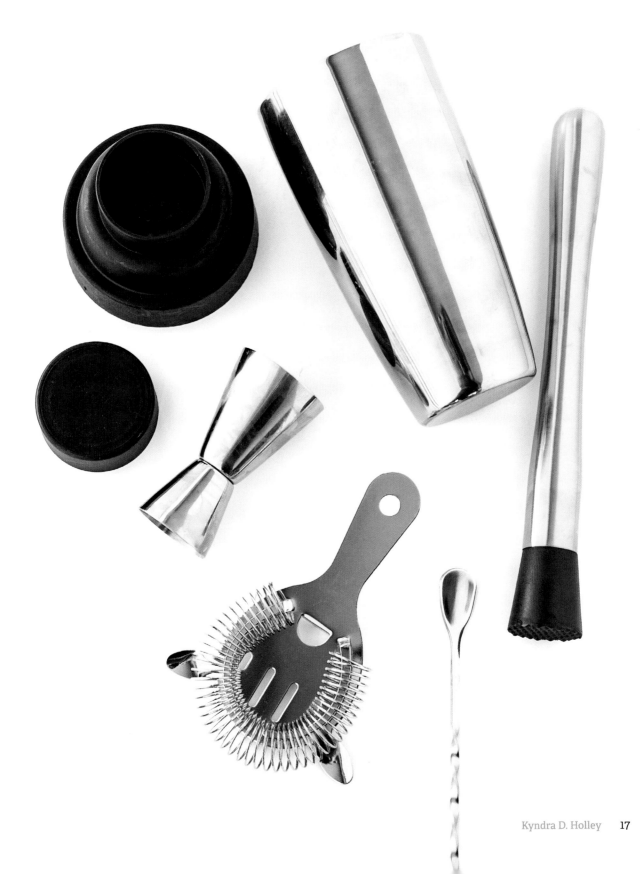

Stocking Your Low-Carb Home Bar

Here are the bar supplies that I stock most often and are used to make the recipes in this book.

SPIRITS, WINES, AND LIQUEURS

Dry red wine   Dry white wine   Gin (dry)   Homemade Coffee Liqueur (page 166)   Homemade Irish Cream Liqueur (page 164)   Rum (white, spiced, dark)   Sparkling wine   Tequila (silver)   Vermouth (dry and sweet)   Vodka   Whiskey   Irish Whiskey

GLASSWARE

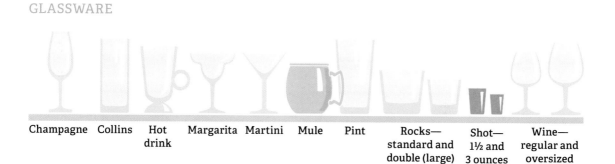

Champagne   Collins   Hot drink   Margarita   Martini   Mule   Pint   Rocks—standard and double (large)   Shot—1½ and 3 ounces (large)   Wine—regular and oversized

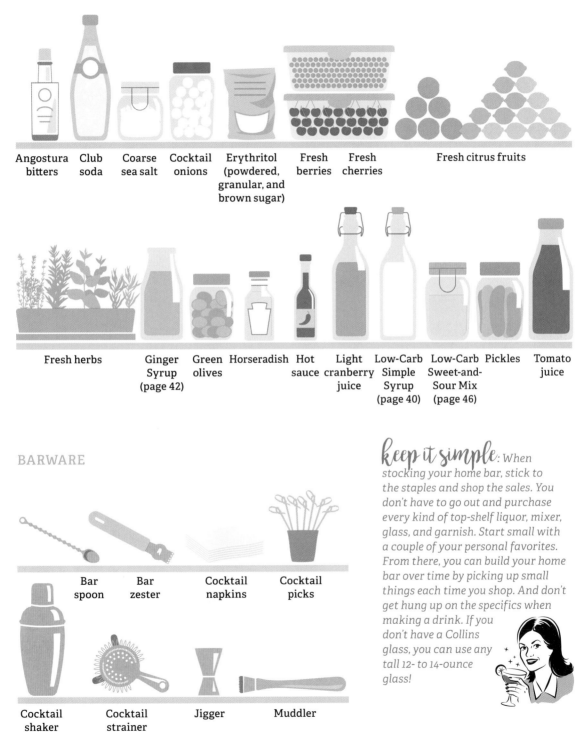

Angostura bitters

Club soda

Coarse sea salt

Cocktail onions

Erythritol (powdered, granular, and brown sugar)

Fresh berries

Fresh cherries

Fresh citrus fruits

Fresh herbs

Ginger Syrup (page 42)

Green olives

Horseradish

Hot sauce

Light cranberry juice

Low-Carb Simple Syrup (page 40)

Low-Carb Sweet-and-Sour Mix (page 46)

Pickles

Tomato juice

BARWARE

Bar spoon

Bar zester

Cocktail napkins

Cocktail picks

Cocktail shaker

Cocktail strainer

Jigger

Muddler

keep it simple: When stocking your home bar, stick to the staples and shop the sales. You don't have to go out and purchase every kind of top-shelf liquor, mixer, glass, and garnish. Start small with a couple of your personal favorites. From there, you can build your home bar over time by picking up small things each time you shop. And don't get hung up on the specifics when making a drink. If you don't have a Collins glass, you can use any tall 12- to 14-ounce glass!

Fruit-and-Herb Pairings

For nearly two centuries, bartenders everywhere have been pushing the limits of creativity and imagination in mastering the craft of the cocktail, from simple and timeless cocktails, like the martini and Manhattan, to more jazzed-up modern cocktails, like the Lavender Ginny (page 90) and the Raspberry Mint Sparkler (page 132).

But these days, bartenders are borrowing more and more from the kitchen in order to redefine the very nature of the cocktail. Why use sugary fruit juices and sodas when you can create dynamic, tantalizing flavor profiles by pairing fresh fruits and herbs?

The guides on the next two pages will teach you how to masterfully pair fresh fruits and herbs with a variety of different liquors to enhance their flavors and make perfectly balanced cocktails.

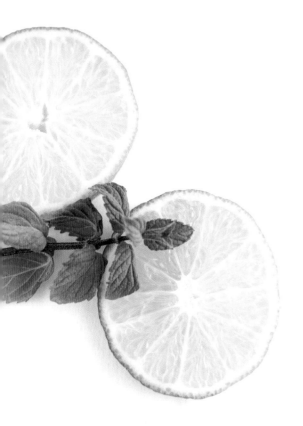

tip: For all the drink recipes and fruit-and-herb pairings in this book, fresh fruit is always recommended unless otherwise specified. Not only will using fresh fruit provide the best flavor, but it will also ensure that you are not unintentionally consuming added sugars, which are sometimes found in frozen or canned fruits. Additionally, maraschino cherries should never be used in place of fresh cherries because they are full of added sugars and artificial ingredients.

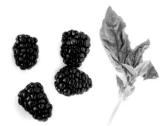

Blackberry and basil

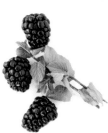

Blackberry and mint

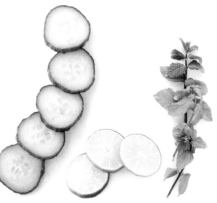

Cucumber, lime, and mint

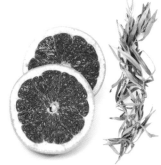

Grapefruit and tarragon

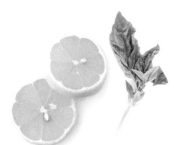

Lemon and basil

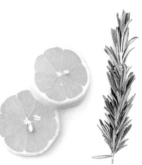

Lemon and rosemary

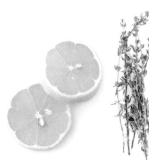

Lemon and thyme

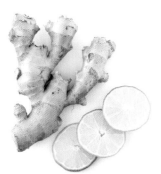

Lime and ginger

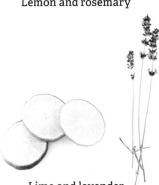

Lime and lavender

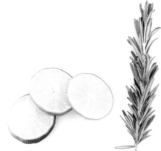

Lime and rosemary

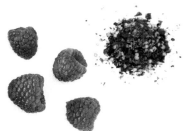

Raspberry and
red pepper flakes

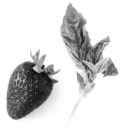

Strawberry and basil

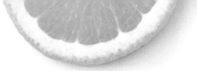

Here are some other great pairings to try once you feel comfortable enough to start experimenting with cocktail creations of your own:

FRUITS AND HERBS	FLAVOR PROFILE	GOES WELL WITH
Strawberry, cucumber, and thyme	Sweet and clean	Vodka or gin
Cucumber, lemon, and rosemary	Clean and earthy	Vodka or gin
Blackberry, lemon, and cilantro	Tart and spicy	White rum or vodka
Blackberry and sage	Tart yet refreshing	Whiskey or gin
Strawberry, lemon, and ginger	Sweet and spicy	White rum or vodka
Strawberry, lemon, and rosemary	Sweet and refreshing, with earthy undertones	Gin or vodka
Ginger, cinnamon, and vanilla	Warm and spicy	Whiskey
Lemon, mint, and ginger	Tart, herbaceous, and spicy	White rum or vodka
Lemon, mint, and lavender	Aromatic and fresh	White rum or vodka
Blueberry and rosemary	Sweet and earthy	Whiskey or vodka
Strawberry and tarragon	Bittersweet	Tequila
Cherry and ginger	Tangy, with a touch of spice	Whiskey
Cranberry, orange, and cinnamon	Seasonal flavors of fall	Whiskey or brandy
Orange and turmeric	Sweet and smoky	Tequila
Grapefruit and parsley	Clean, tart, and refreshing	Tequila or vodka

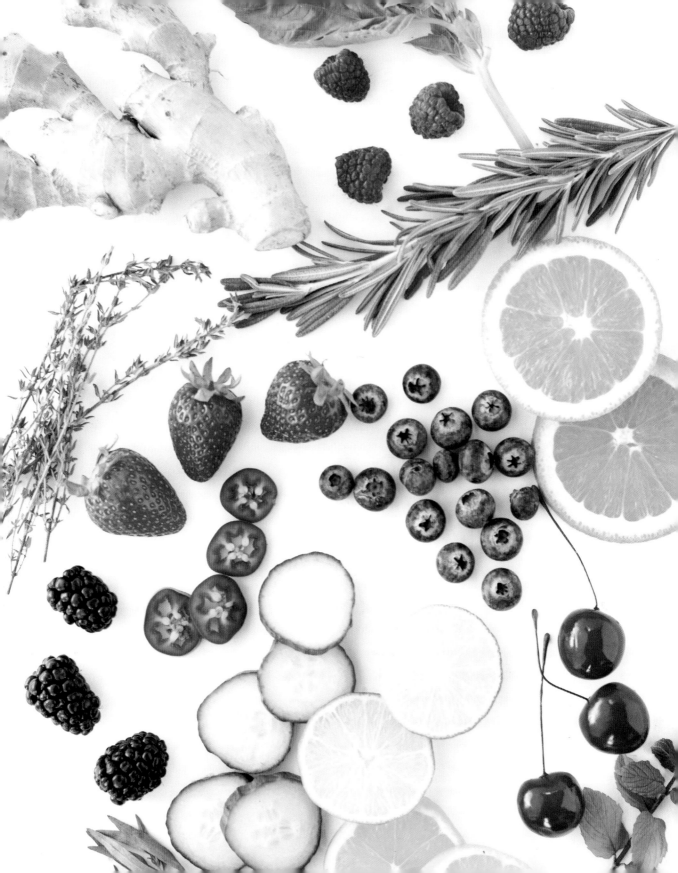

My Top Ten Tips for Hosting the Perfect Cocktail Party

So you've got recipes for low-carb drinks and party foods. Your home bar is stocked and ready to go. You've learned how to make cocktails like a master mixologist. You are a pro at fruit-and-herb pairings, and you've got the bartending vernacular down like it's in your ancestry. Now what? It's time to put together everything you have learned and throw the most amazing low-carb cocktail party anyone has ever seen. Here are my best tips for hosting an unforgettable event that people will be talking about for years to come.

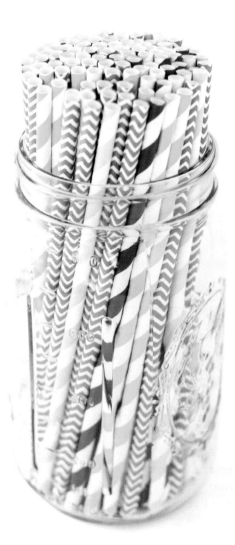

1.
Gauge the Guest Count

First, decide how many people you want to invite. Everything else hinges upon the guest count. Make sure that you do not invite more people than your space can reasonably accommodate. You want your guests to be comfortable, and you want to be able to provide enough food and drink for each guest, with a little extra for any surprise appearances. Additionally, you want to be able to engage with each of your guests, and keeping the guest list short will allow you to do so. Decide ahead of time whether each guest is allowed to bring a plus-one and note it on the invitation so that you are not surprised by more guests than you planned for.

2.
Think about a Theme

It is important that your guests know what to expect. Is this a casual get-together, or is it more formal in nature? Is there something specific they should wear? You would hate to host a formal event and have guests show up in togas. Have fun with it. Host a low-key party with a simple theme and encourage your guests to get creative with homemade costumes. You can even give out prizes for the best costumes. Need help selecting a theme? Here are some of my favorites: the eighties, prom night, television and movie characters, pajama party, Hawaiian tiki, murder mystery, hair bands, mobsters, and famous couples. The possibilities are truly endless.

3.
Don't Break the Bank

Once you have decided on the guest count and the theme of your party, you can set a budget. Decide how much you are willing to spend for the event and stick to that amount. The budget you set should incorporate everything needed for the entire event— food, drinks, decorations, and so on. If you can't budget it in, you don't need it. Remember, your guests are there to see you, not the decorations.

4.
Plan the Plates

Now that you have established how many people will be attending and how much you are going to spend, it's time to set the food menu. It is not necessary to serve a full-course meal. Passable appetizers and finger foods will do the trick. Just make sure that there is enough food for all your guests to get a fair amount. You don't want them throwing back cocktails on an empty stomach.

5.
Decide the Drinks

Just as you set the food menu, it is important to set the drink menu, too. You want to choose drinks that pair nicely with the flavor profiles of the foods you have selected. For help with pairing food and drinks, refer to the party menus on pages 28 to 33. It is likely that some of your guests will bring drinks to share, but it is best to assume that you will be responsible for supplying all the drinks for your guests unless otherwise noted on the invite.

6.
Perfect the Playlist

Pick the music in advance and have it playing low in the background, without interruptions from commercials. Choose music that is pleasing to most people and blends into the background so that your guests can easily interact and engage with one another without having to raise their voices.

7.
Grab the Games

Whether it is a life-sized backyard Jenga game or a good old-fashioned board game, playing games is a great way to liven up any party. Better yet, consider setting up game stations for people to rotate through over the course of the evening.

8.
Set the Scene

From decorations to lighting, every little decision you make sets the scene for the event. Make sure you have several gathering spaces, with adequate seating for your guests. Avoid harsh lighting and extreme temperatures. Be sure to designate an area for coats, shoes, bags, and other personal belongings.

9.
Entertain with Ease

Don't sweat the small stuff. There may be hiccups, but the chances that anyone will actually notice are very slim. Just be yourself, and work on being present and having a good time. It is a party, after all. If, during the planning stages, it starts to feel like the night might become a little overwhelming for you, don't be afraid to enlist the help of a willing friend. Or cohost the event, splitting the work and costs with another person.

10.
Don't Allow Drunk Driving

Your guests are in your care, and even the smartest and most responsible adults sometimes need someone else to be the voice of reason. As one drink turns into two, then three, then four, the rational brain may no longer be in control. Hey, we've all been there! Let your guests know that there is no shame in admitting they have overindulged. The only shame is in taking the risk of harming themselves or others. Don't be afraid to step up and let overindulgers know that you are not comfortable with them driving. Do your best to provide a place where they can safely wait it out, or arrange for a ride home.

Low-Carb Party Planning

Whether you are hosting a game night, getting together with friends to watch the big game, or having people over for a summertime cookout, the food-and-drink pairings on the following pages have you covered. Each menu does the thinking for you, listing everything you need to host the most fabulous and unforgettable keto gathering ever. The accompanying shopping lists tell you which ingredients you'll need to have on hand.

Visit peaceloveandlowcarb.com for printable grocery lists with exact amounts of everything you'll need for each of these low-carb party menus. Be sure to check your fridge and pantry before heading to the grocery store, as there is a good chance that you will already have many of the staple ingredients on hand. Happy party planning!

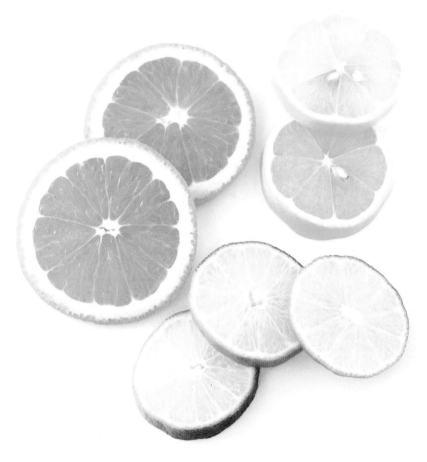

WINTER WONDERLAND

Eats

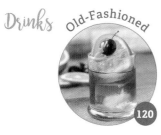

Teriyaki Steak Bites — 194

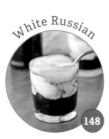

Crispy Baked Garlic-Parmesan Wings — 184

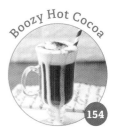

Barbecue Cocktail Sausages — 176

Drinks

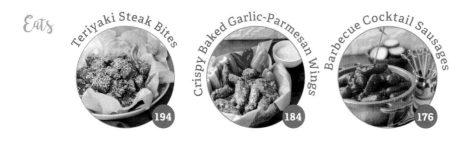

Old-Fashioned — 120

White Russian — 148

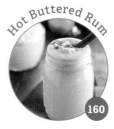

Hot Buttered Rum — 160

Boozy Hot Cocoa — 154

Shopping List

Alcohol
Irish whiskey
Spiced rum
Vodka
Whiskey

Dairy/Eggs
Butter
Grated Parmesan cheese
Heavy cream

Meat/Poultry/Seafood
Chicken wings
Smoked beef cocktail sausages
Steak

Pantry/Condiments/Spices
Angostura bitters
Apple cider vinegar
Baking powder
Coconut aminos
Espresso granules
Garlic powder
Liquid smoke
Olive oil
Onion powder
Powdered erythritol
Pure almond extract
Pure vanilla extract
Sesame seeds

Sugar-free, low-carb hot cocoa
Tomato sauce
Unseasoned rice vinegar
Unsweetened cocoa powder
Xanthan gum

Produce
Fresh flat-leaf parsley
Fresh ginger
Garlic
Green onions
Lemon
Orange

Optional
Bibb lettuce
Brown sugar erythritol
Fresh cherries
Sugar-free dark chocolate

GAME NIGHT

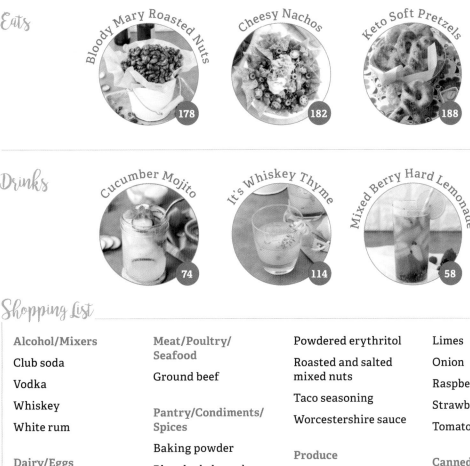

Eats

Bloody Mary Roasted Nuts 178

Cheesy Nachos 182

Keto Soft Pretzels 188

Drinks

Cucumber Mojito 74

It's Whiskey Thyme 114

Mixed Berry Hard Lemonade 58

Shopping List

Alcohol/Mixers
Club soda
Vodka
Whiskey
White rum

Dairy/Eggs
Butter
Cream cheese
Eggs
Grated Parmesan cheese
Sharp cheddar cheese
Shredded low-moisture, part-skim mozzarella cheese
Sour cream

Meat/Poultry/Seafood
Ground beef

Pantry/Condiments/Spices
Baking powder
Blanched almond flour
Celery salt
Chili powder
Coarse sea salt
Garlic powder
Granular erythritol
Ground cumin
Hot sauce
Onion powder

Powdered erythritol
Roasted and salted mixed nuts
Taco seasoning
Worcestershire sauce

Produce
Blackberries
Blueberries
English cucumbers
Fresh ginger
Fresh mint
Fresh thyme
Guacamole
Jalapeño pepper
Lemons

Limes
Onion
Raspberries
Strawberries
Tomato

Canned/Jarred Goods
Sliced black olives
Tomato paste

Optional
Fresh cilantro

SUMMER LOVIN'

Eats

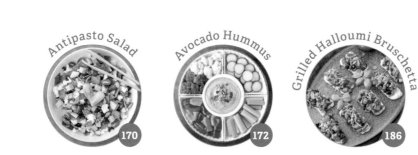

Antipasto Salad — 170

Avocado Hummus — 172

Grilled Halloumi Bruschetta — 186

Drinks

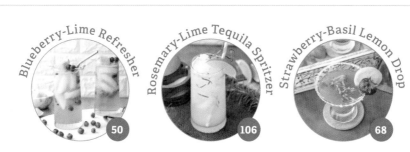

Blueberry-Lime Refresher — 50

Rosemary-Lime Tequila Spritzer — 106

Strawberry-Basil Lemon Drop — 68

Shopping List

Alcohol/Mixers

Club soda

Silver tequila

Vodka

Dairy/Eggs

Grated Parmesan cheese

Halloumi cheese

Sharp cheddar cheese

Meat/Poultry/Seafood

Pepperoni slices

Salami slices

Pantry/Condiments/Spices

Avocado oil

Balsamic vinegar

Granular erythritol

Ground cumin

Powdered erythritol

Roasted tahini

Produce

Avocado

Blueberries

Cauliflower

Cucumber

Fresh basil

Fresh rosemary

Garlic

Grape tomatoes

Lemons

Limes

Strawberries

Tomato

Zucchini

Canned/Jarred Goods

Capers

Kalamata olives

Mayonnaise

Sliced black olives

BRUNCH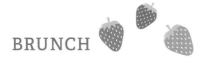

Eats

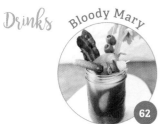
Bacon and Blue Cheese Deviled Eggs — 174

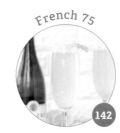
Grilled Halloumi Bruschetta — 186

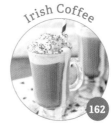
Pork Belly BLTC Stacks — 192

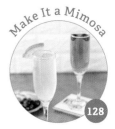

Drinks

Bloody Mary — 62

French 75 — 142

Irish Coffee — 162

Make It a Mimosa — 128

Shopping List

Alcohol/Mixers
Champagne
Dry gin
Irish whiskey
Light cranberry juice
Vodka

Dairy/Eggs
Blue cheese crumbles
Eggs
Grated Parmesan cheese
Halloumi cheese
Heavy cream
Sharp cheddar cheese

Meat/Poultry/Seafood
Bacon
Precooked pork belly

Pantry/Condiments/Spices
Avocado oil
Balsamic vinegar
Celery salt
Coffee
Dried minced onions
Garlic powder
Hot sauce
Instant espresso granules
Powdered erythritol

Pure almond extract
Pure vanilla extract
Unsweetened cocoa powder
Worcestershire sauce

Produce
Fresh basil
Fresh chives
Fresh dill weed
Garlic
Grapefruit
Grape tomatoes
Lemons
Raspberries
Romaine lettuce

Strawberries
Tomato

Canned/Jarred Goods
Capers
Dill pickles
Horseradish
Mayonnaise
Pitted Kalamata olives
Tomato juice

Optional
Fresh cranberries
Pickled vegetables
Sugar-free dark chocolate

GIRLS' NIGHT

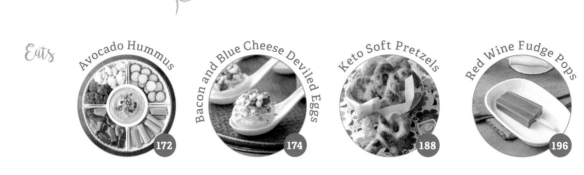

Eats

Avocado Hummus — 172

Bacon and Blue Cheese Deviled Eggs — 174

Keto Soft Pretzels — 188

Red Wine Fudge Pops — 196

Drinks

Cosmopolitan — 52

Lady in Red — 126

Mixed Berry Prosecco Slushie — 130

Shopping List

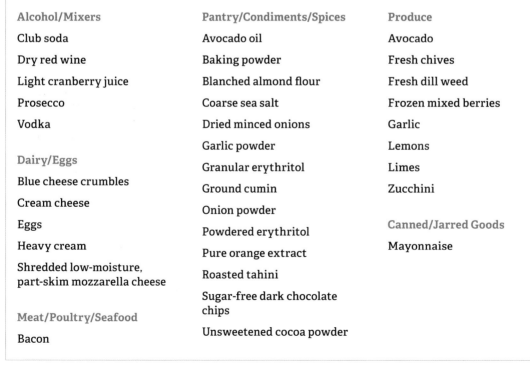

Alcohol/Mixers

Club soda

Dry red wine

Light cranberry juice

Prosecco

Vodka

Dairy/Eggs

Blue cheese crumbles

Cream cheese

Eggs

Heavy cream

Shredded low-moisture, part-skim mozzarella cheese

Meat/Poultry/Seafood

Bacon

Pantry/Condiments/Spices

Avocado oil

Baking powder

Blanched almond flour

Coarse sea salt

Dried minced onions

Garlic powder

Granular erythritol

Ground cumin

Onion powder

Powdered erythritol

Pure orange extract

Roasted tahini

Sugar-free dark chocolate chips

Unsweetened cocoa powder

Produce

Avocado

Fresh chives

Fresh dill weed

Frozen mixed berries

Garlic

Lemons

Limes

Zucchini

Canned/Jarred Goods

Mayonnaise

GUYS' NIGHT

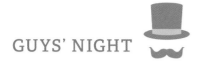

Eats

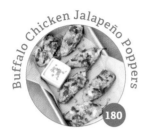
Buffalo Chicken Jalapeño Poppers **180**

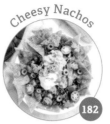
Cheesy Nachos **182**

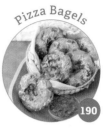
Pizza Bagels **190**

Drinks

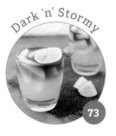
Dark 'n' Stormy **73**

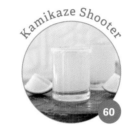
Kamikaze Shooter **60**

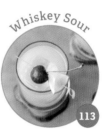
Whiskey Sour **113**

Shopping List

Alcohol/Mixers
Club soda
Dark rum
Vodka
Whiskey

Dairy/Eggs
Blue cheese crumbles
Cream cheese
Eggs
Grated Parmesan cheese
Sharp cheddar cheese
Shredded low-moisture, part-skim mozzarella cheese
Sour cream

Meat/Poultry/Seafood
Bacon
Ground beef
Ground chicken
Pepperoni slices

Pantry/Condiments/Spices
Baking powder
Blanched almond flour
Buffalo wing sauce
Chili powder
Coarse sea salt
Dried oregano leaves
Garlic powder

Granular erythritol
Ground cumin
Italian seasoning
Onion powder
Powdered erythritol
Pure orange extract
Taco seasoning

Produce
Fresh ginger
Green onions
Guacamole
Jalapeño peppers
Lemons
Limes

Onion
Tomato

Canned/Jarred Goods
Low-carb pizza sauce (or make homemade; see the recipe on peaceloveandlowcarb.com)
Sliced black olives

Optional
Fresh cherries
Fresh cilantro

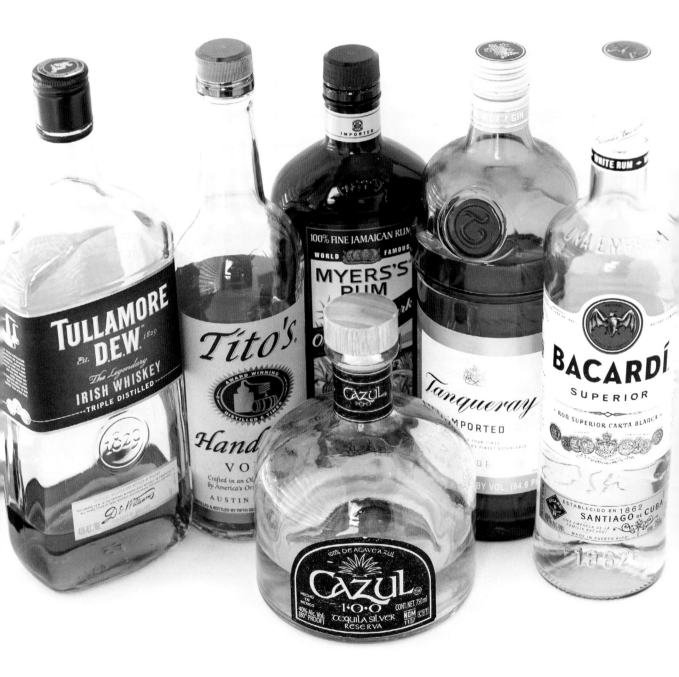

Hangover Hacks

It happens to the best of us: You meet a friend for happy hour, and one drink turns into two. Before you know it, two drinks turn into three. Then, in the blink of an eye, happy hour has come and gone and you are sipping on a full-priced cocktail with a full-on buzz vibrating through you. While I don't believe there is truly any magic elixir that can banish the booze blues, these tips might make the day after a little more bearable—or, better yet, keep you from getting a hangover at all.

THE NIGHT OF

Fill Up on Fat

Contrary to popular hangover belief, it's actually more beneficial to eat a big high-fat meal *before* you drink than to eat it the next day, when you are already nursing a hangover. Additionally, eating something—*anything*—before you drink is always a good idea, as having food in your stomach will help to slow down the rate of alcohol absorption.

Hydrate, Hydrate, Hydrate

Alcohol is a diuretic, which means that it will make you urinate more than if you were drinking an equal amount of water. This excess urination opens you up to thirst and dehydration. Dehydration can bring on headaches, dry mouth, and fatigue. Drinking water between alcoholic drinks will not only help keep you hydrated but also slow down the rate at which you are drinking cocktails.

Keep It Clear

Stick to clear liquors. Colorless alcohols like white rum and gin contain low levels of congeners, toxic chemicals formed in small amounts when alcohol is produced. Vodka contains almost none at all. Two of the liquors with higher levels of congeners are tequila and whiskey. Higher levels of congeners increase the chances of getting a hangover and the intensity of the hangover. When in doubt, keep it clear!

THE NEXT DAY

Hydrate, Hydrate, Hydrate

Can you tell that I am serious about this one? I've stressed the importance of staying hydrated the night of, but it is just as important to continue focusing on hydration the next day. Drinking a lot of water is perhaps the single best thing you can do for your body after a night of drinking. Water is the magical elixir that keeps your body alive and thriving.

Eat an Eggcellent Breakfast

Hangovers are sometimes associated with low blood sugar, so eating a healthy breakfast as soon as you rise can help restore normal blood sugar levels. Eggs make for a great hangover breakfast because they are packed with amino acids like cysteine and taurine. Taurine helps boost liver function, and chances are your liver could use a good boost after a night of overindulging. Cysteine helps break down acetaldehyde, the headache-inducing chemical that is left over after the liver has broken down the alcohol.

Have a Pickleback (page 122)

Science calls brine a hangover cure. Well, it says that the acetic acid in vinegar is an antidiuretic that contains electrolytes and absorbs salt. Pair it with the "hair of the dog," and you've got yourself a perfect breakfast cocktail. Be careful, though—while it might make you feel better temporarily, the hair of the dog might just come back to bite you.

Sip on Gut-Healing Bone Broth

Bone broth has some amazing health-promoting properties. It is a great source of amino acids, collagen, gelatin, and minerals—all things you need more of after a night of drinking. It helps promote a healthy gut and aids in proper digestion. It also helps reduce inflammation and support healthy immune function. It is a great addition to your everyday routine, but it is especially helpful after overindulging.

Replenish Your Electrolytes

You have likely heard this one a million times, but have you ever really dug into just what it is you are replenishing? Some of the electrolytes that the human body needs to survive are sodium, potassium, calcium bicarbonate, magnesium chloride, hydrogen phosphate, and hydrogen carbonate. Each one serves a different function in the body, but sodium is perhaps the most important after a night of drinking: it regulates the body's use of water. So how can you replenish these electrolytes? Skip the sugary sports drinks and replenish electrolytes naturally through low-carb real foods. For sodium, put a pinch of salt in your drinking water. Foods like pumpkin seeds, peanut butter, spinach, and almonds are great sources of magnesium. Coconut water is a great source of potassium, magnesium, and sodium.

Get Bendy with Yoga

Yoga helps calm the central nervous system, improves circulation, aids in digestion, resets the endocrine system, and helps release toxins from the body. These are all things that will help bring your body back into a state of harmony after a night of drinking. Some great poses if you have a hangover are child's pose, corpse pose, cat-cow pose, supine spinal twist, supported fetal position, and upward-facing dog pose. Stick to a gentle yoga practice, and avoid hot yoga during a hangover, as it can further dehydrate the body.

Rest, Rest, Rest

Your body probably feels like it just went through a war. Honor it by resting up and not overexerting yourself. Take a nap, binge-watch your favorite show, and just take things easy. The more you give your body a chance to recover, the faster it will bounce back.

Kick Up the Caffeine

This one comes with very mixed reviews. Many people will tell you to skip the coffee after a night of drinking, while others will advise you to drink up. Like a lot of these hangover hacks, what works for some might not work for others. But if you are an everyday coffee drinker, passing on the bean juice isn't going to do anything but give you caffeine withdrawal and perhaps an even worse headache. That being said, maybe limit it to one cup until you are feeling like yourself again.

Take a Quality Multivitamin

I hope you are already taking a quality multivitamin daily, but replenishing essential vitamins and minerals is especially important after a night of drinking.

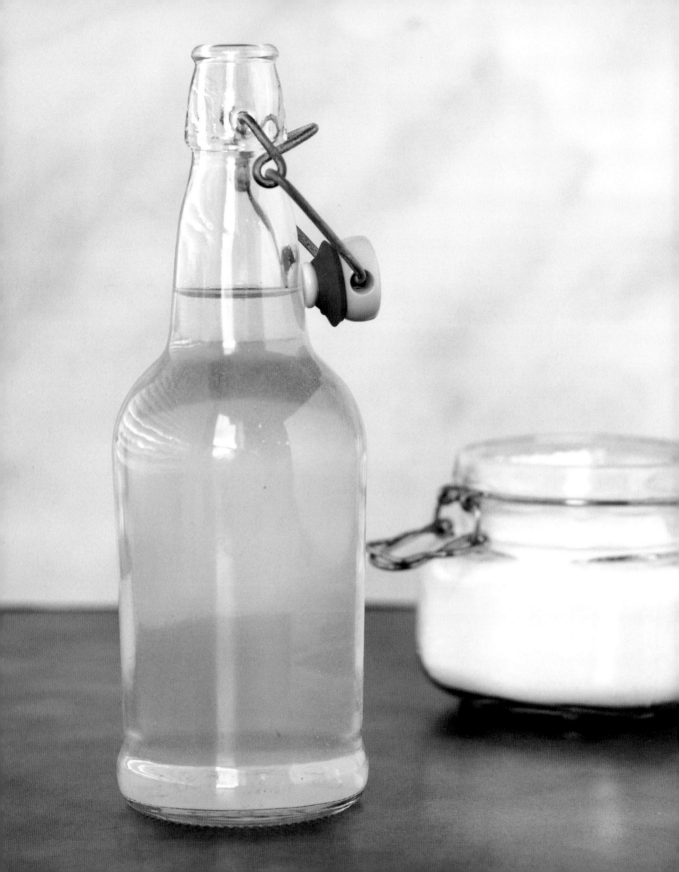

CHAPTER 1

MIXERS AND OTHER
Fun Stuff

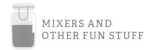

Low-Carb Simple Syrup

Simple syrup is the main sweetener for cocktails of all shapes and sizes. It isn't just simple by name; it is also simple to prepare. It is simply (pun intended) sugar, or in this case the natural sweetener erythritol, heated and dissolved in water to give it a sweet taste and a smooth texture.

Makes 20 ounces (1 ounce per serving)

2 cups granular or powdered erythritol

1 cup water

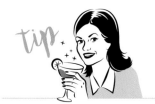

If the mixture starts to separate in the refrigerator and the erythritol begins to crystallize, simply reheat the simple syrup on the stovetop until it dissolves again.

1 In a medium saucepan over medium-high heat, combine the erythritol and water. Bring to a boil, then reduce the heat to low and cook, stirring constantly, until the erythritol has dissolved, about 5 minutes.

2 Remove the pan from the heat and allow to cool, then transfer the syrup to a 32-ounce mason jar. Store in the refrigerator for up to 1 month.

. . . .

If you do not want to make an entire batch of simple syrup, you can simply use powdered erythritol in the recipes throughout this book. With its ultrafine powdery texture, it dissolves into cocktails without leaving a grainy texture. Because this simple syrup is made with a 2:1 ratio of sweetener to water, you can substitute an equal amount of powdered erythritol.

¼ ounce simple syrup = 1½ teaspoons powdered erythritol

⅓ ounce simple syrup = 2 teaspoons powdered erythritol

½ ounce simple syrup = 1 tablespoon powdered erythritol

¾ ounce simple syrup = 1 tablespoon + 1½ teaspoons powdered erythritol

1 ounce simple syrup = 2 tablespoons powdered erythritol

. . . .

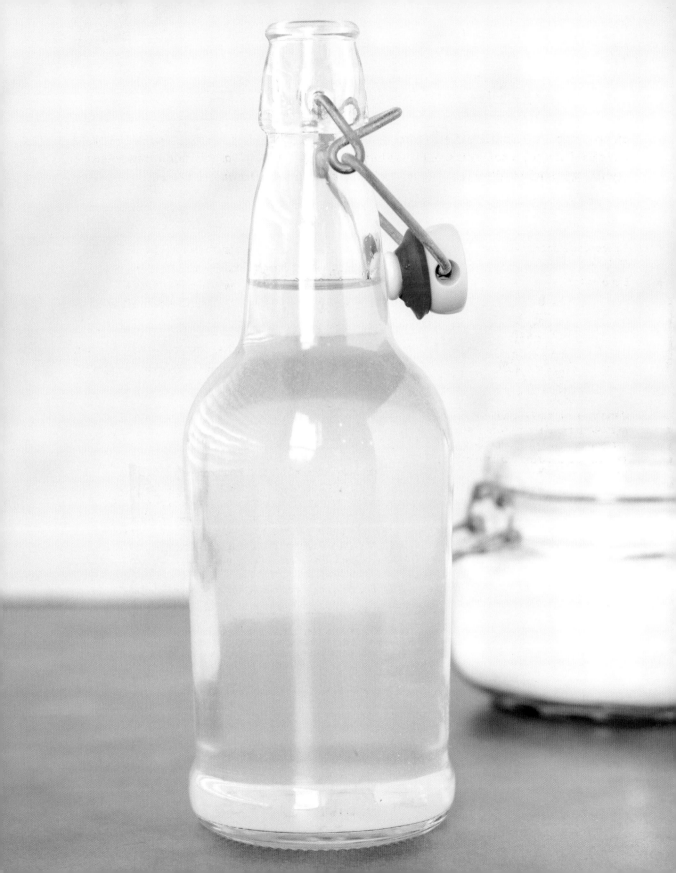

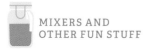

Ginger Syrup

Ginger somehow manages to be both sweet and spicy, making it a great pairing for a wide variety of cocktails. This syrup is very concentrated in flavor—a little goes a long way. Try mixing 2 ounces into a large glass of ice-cold club soda for a delicious and refreshing mocktail.

Makes 16 ounces (2 ounces per serving)

2 cups water

½ cup granular erythritol

⅓ cup grated fresh ginger

1 Combine the water, erythritol, and ginger in a small saucepan. Bring to a boil over high heat, then reduce the heat to low and simmer for 20 minutes, until the sugar has dissolved and the liquid has begun to thicken.

2 Remove from the heat and let the mixture cool, then strain through a sieve to remove the ginger pulp.

3 Transfer the syrup to a pint-sized mason jar with a lid. Store in the refrigerator for up to 2 weeks.

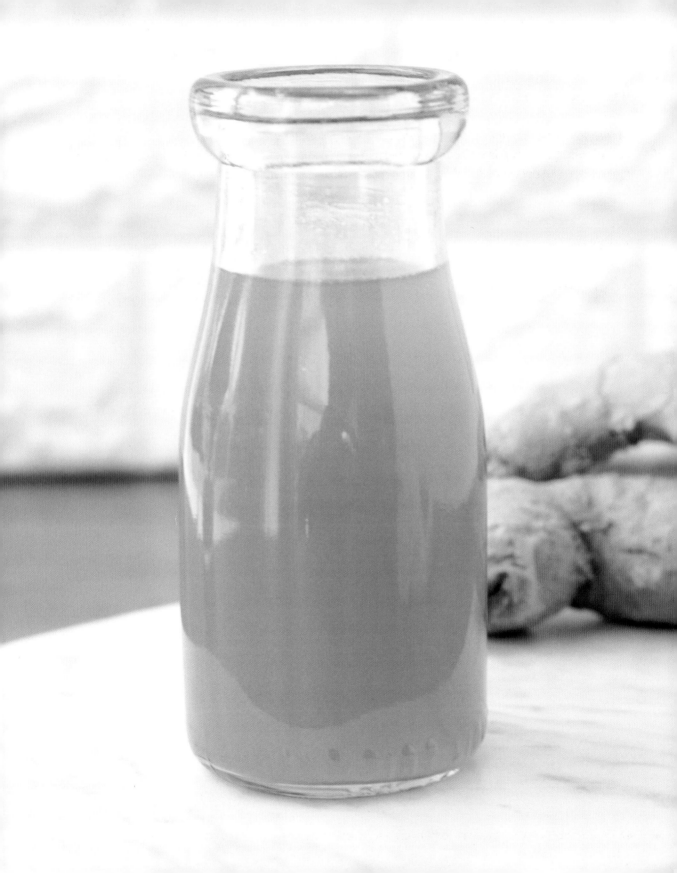

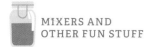

Bloody Mary Mix

Whether mixed with vodka for a Bloody Mary (page 62) or with tequila for a Bloody Maria (page 98)—or even all on its own—this mix is the perfect blend of spicy and zesty.

Makes 28 ounces (4 ounces per serving)

24 ounces tomato juice

2 tablespoons dill pickle juice

2 tablespoons fresh lemon juice

2 tablespoons Worcestershire sauce

2 teaspoons prepared horseradish

2 teaspoons hot sauce, such as Tapatio or Cholula

1 teaspoon celery salt

1 teaspoon garlic powder

1 teaspoon fine sea salt

¼ teaspoon ground black pepper

Combine all the ingredients in a 32-ounce wide-mouthed mason jar. Cap and shake to combine. Store in the refrigerator for up to 2 weeks.

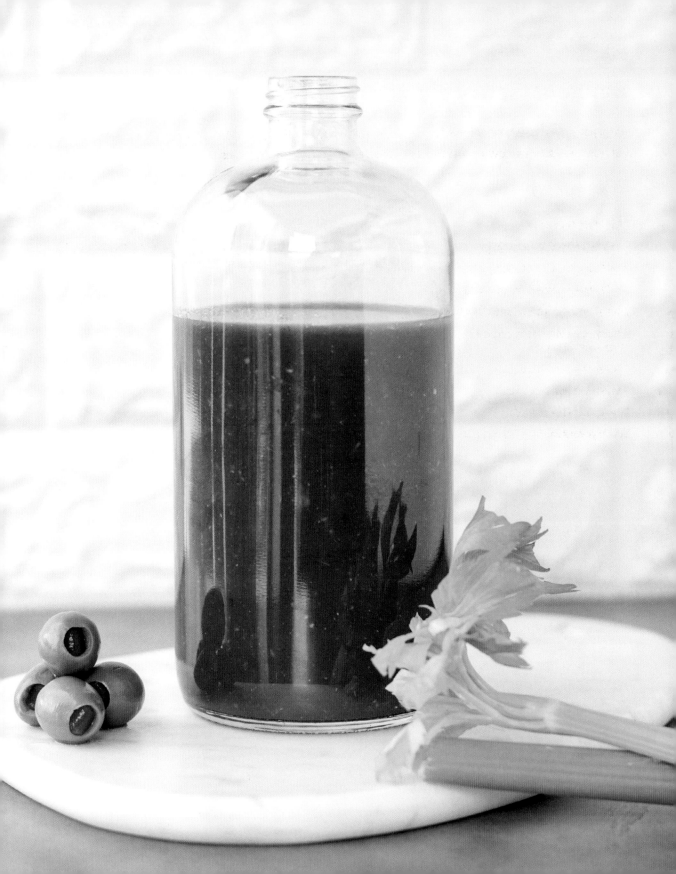

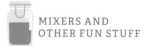

MIXERS AND
OTHER FUN STUFF

NET CARBS
2.1g

Low-Carb Sweet-and-Sour Mix

A mainstay in modern mixology, sweet-and-sour mix is the quintessential drink mixer. It is one of the few mixers that works with multiple liquors: it's great not only with gin, rum, and vodka but also with whiskey and tequila. You might be surprised at just how easy it is to make your own low-carb sweet-and-sour mix.

Makes 32 ounces (2 ounces per serving)

1 cup fresh lemon juice

1 cup fresh lime juice

1 cup water

1 cup powdered erythritol

Combine all the ingredients in a 32-ounce wide-mouthed mason jar. Cap and shake to combine. Store in the refrigerator for up to 2 weeks. Shake well before using.

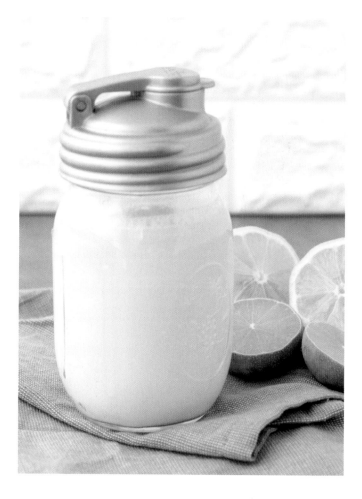

46   CALORIES: 7 | FAT: 0.1g | PROTEIN: 0.2g | TOTAL CARBS: 2.3g | DIETARY FIBER: 0.2g | NET CARBS: 2.1g | ERYTHRITOL: 12g

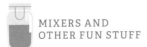

Fresh Whipped Cream

There is nothing in the world quite like fresh whipped cream. Considering how simple it is to make, it is a wonder anyone would ever use the store-bought variety. This recipe is best when made for immediate use.

Makes 2½ cups (2 tablespoons per serving)

1 cup heavy cream

1 tablespoon plus 1 teaspoon powdered erythritol

1 teaspoon pure vanilla extract

Combine all the ingredients in a large mixing bowl. Using a hand mixer, whip until the cream forms stiff peaks, 3 to 4 minutes.

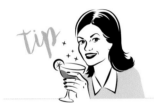

For a chocolate variation, add 1 tablespoon of unsweetened cocoa powder and increase the erythritol to 2 tablespoons.

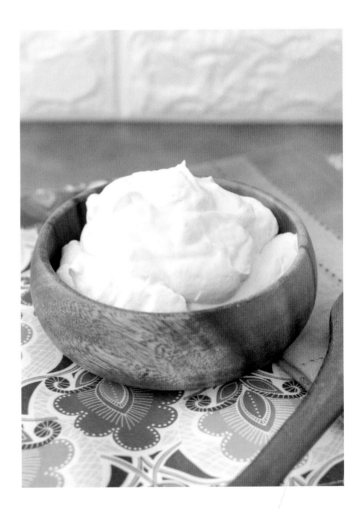

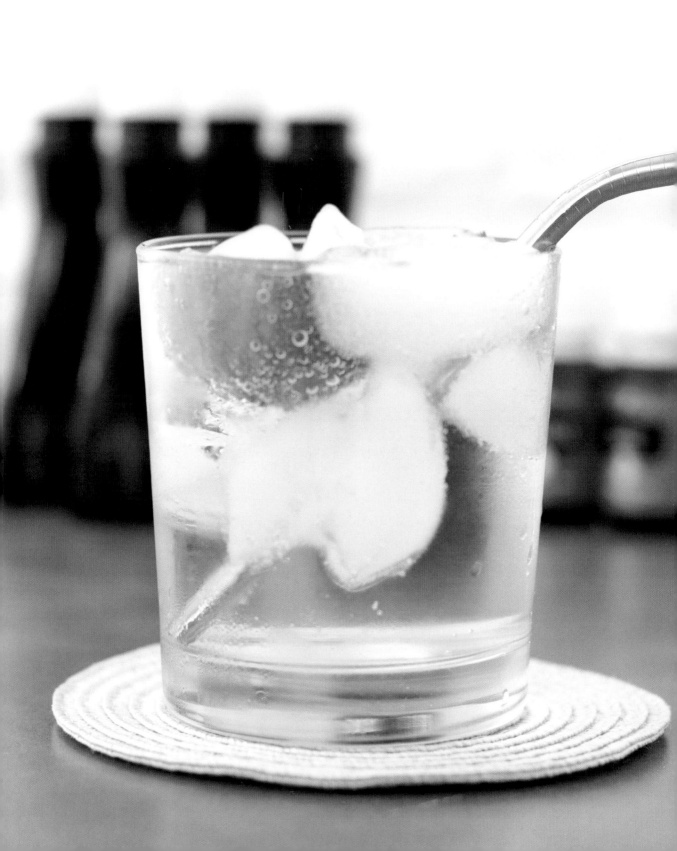

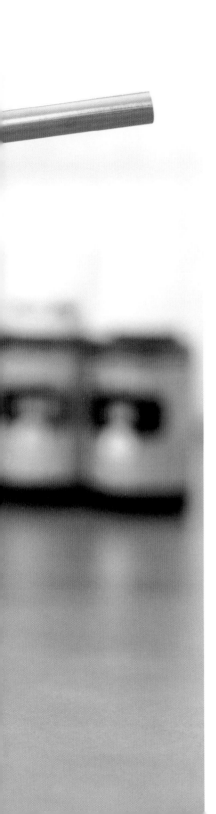

VODKA
drinks

Blueberry-Lime Refresher

Refreshing, indeed! This is one of those beverages that can easily get away from you. It tastes delicious and goes down easy. One drink turns into two and two turns into three as you visit with friends about the week you all just had. Before you know it, you have that familiar floating sensation of a summertime buzz.

Makes 1 drink

½ lime, cut into 4 wedges, divided

¼ ounce Low-Carb Simple Syrup (page 40)

2 tablespoons blueberries, plus more for garnish

1½ ounces vodka

5 ounces club soda

1   Fill a pint-sized glass with ice.

2   Put 3 of the lime wedges, the simple syrup, and the blueberries in a cocktail shaker. Muddle until the fruit is crushed and has released its liquid.

3   Add the vodka to the cocktail shaker. Cap and shake vigorously.

4   Strain the contents of the cocktail shaker into the ice-filled glass. Top with the club soda and stir.

5   Garnish with the remaining lime wedge and extra blueberries.

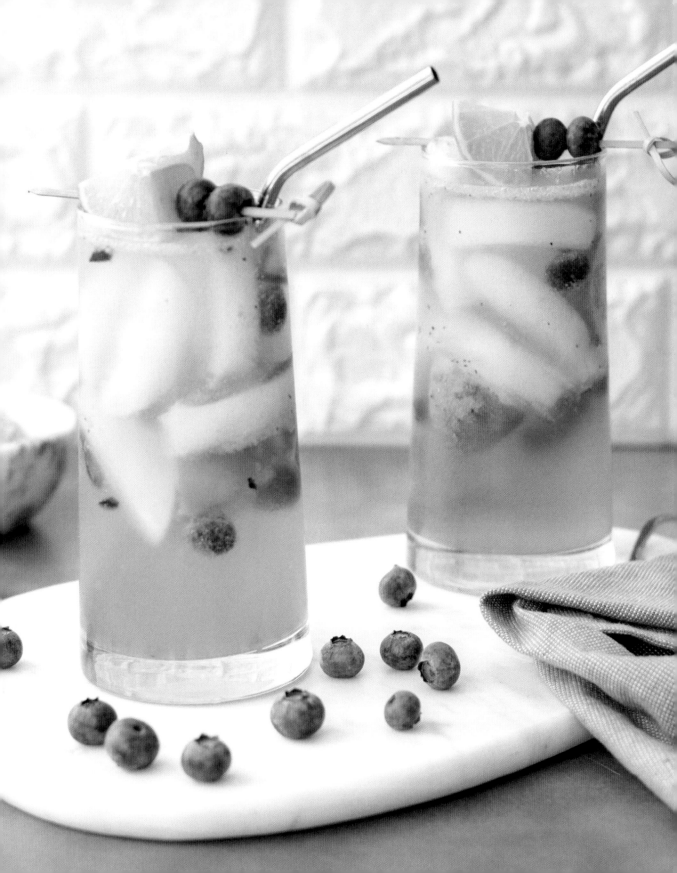

VODKA
DRINKS

NET CARBS
3g

Cosmopolitan

Although the Cosmopolitan has been around for ages, it soared in popularity in the late 1990s when Carrie Bradshaw and her Sex and the City crew gave this drink a cult following. This classic still graces happy hour menus everywhere and continues to be a favorite. With this low-carb version, you can sip on Cosmos with your friends without worrying about your waistline.

Makes 1 drink

2 ounces vodka

1½ ounces light cranberry juice

½ ounce fresh lime juice

¼ ounce Low-Carb Simple Syrup (page 40)

2 drops of pure orange extract

Lime wheel, for garnish

1 Fill a cocktail shaker with ice. Add the vodka, cranberry juice, lime juice, simple syrup, and orange extract. Cap and shake vigorously.

2 Strain the contents of the cocktail shaker into a chilled martini glass and garnish with a lime wheel.

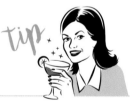

tip

If you have already purchased dried lavender buds for the Lavender Ginny (page 90), try adding ½ teaspoon to this Cosmo recipe for a floral and fruity variation.

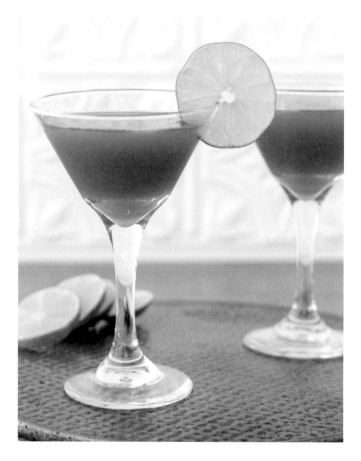

52   CALORIES: 151 | FAT: 0 | PROTEIN: 0 | TOTAL CARBS: 3g | DIETARY FIBER: 0 | NET CARBS: 3g | ERYTHRITOL: 6g

Vodka Soda

I went back and forth about including so simple a drink in this book, but then I realized that it might just be getting overlooked. This is perhaps the easiest cocktail to spruce up to suit your own personal tastes. I like to take a basic Vodka Soda and flavor it with different extracts or pure essential oils. Adding a couple drops of grapefruit essential oil is my favorite way to enjoy this simple low-carb cocktail.

Makes 1 drink

1½ ounces vodka

3 ounces club soda

2 lime wedges

1 Fill a rocks glass with ice. Pour the vodka over the ice and top with the club soda.

2 Squeeze in the lime wedges and stir.

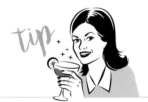

For some other delicious flavor combinations that you can add to this drink, check out the discussion of fruit-and-herb pairings on pages 20 to 22.

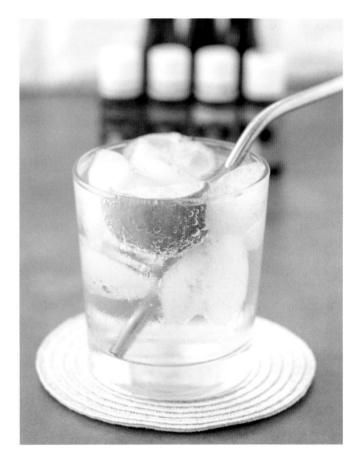

VODKA
DRINKS

NET CARBS
0

Dill Pickle Martini

If you have followed my site over the years or own any of my other books, then you know that I have a serious dill pickle obsession. When I started listing the drinks I wanted to make for this book, a dirty martini was close to the top. But instead of olive juice, which is what traditionally makes a martini "dirty," I knew right away that I wanted to use pickle juice. If you prefer a more traditional dirty martini, substitute olive brine for the pickle juice.

Makes 1 drink

4 ounces vodka

¼ teaspoon dry vermouth (optional; see note)

1½ ounces dill pickle juice

1 Fill a cocktail shaker with ice. Add the vodka, vermouth (if using), and pickle juice. Cap and shake vigorously.

2 Strain the contents of the cocktail shaker into a chilled martini glass. Garnish with a cornichon or a dill pickle spear and any other fun keto-friendly pickled vegetables you have on hand.

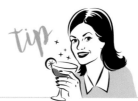

tip

If you prefer gin martinis, this drink is delicious made with gin.

note

Traditional martinis, dirty or otherwise, are made with vermouth. I've made it optional here because I prefer my martinis sans vermouth—and with the pickle brine, you don't really need it anyway.

CALORIES: 282 | FAT: 0 | PROTEIN: 0 | TOTAL CARBS: 0 | DIETARY FIBER: 0 | NET CARBS: 0

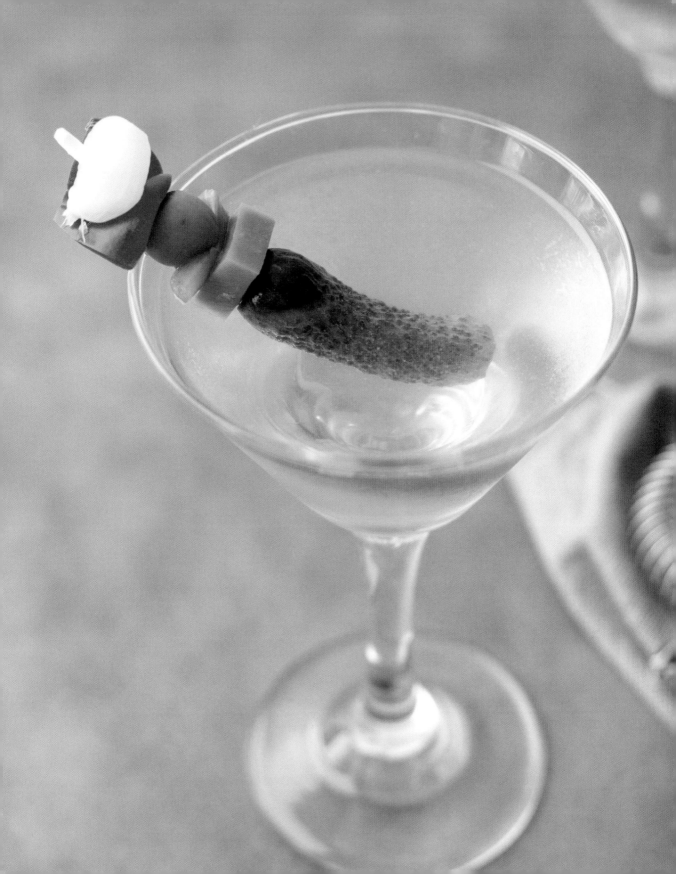

Fruity Boozy Fizzer

This drink just screams summertime to me. Perhaps it is because I created this recipe on a beautiful Pacific Northwest summer day, or maybe it's because it is just so fresh and light tasting. Either way, all I can say is, "Yes, please! I'll have another!"

Makes 1 drink

2 ounces vodka

4 strawberries, hulled and quartered

2 lemon wedges

2 lime wedges

2 ounces Sweet-and-Sour Mix (page 46)

Club soda

1 Put the vodka, strawberries, and lemon and lime wedges in a cocktail shaker. Muddle until the fruits are crushed and have released their juices.

2 Add the sweet-and-sour mix to the cocktail shaker and fill it the rest of the way with ice. Cap and shake vigorously.

3 Pour the contents of the cocktail shaker into a pint-sized glass and top with club soda.

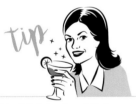

tip

This drink is also delicious with tequila. It tastes like a scratch-made fruity margarita.

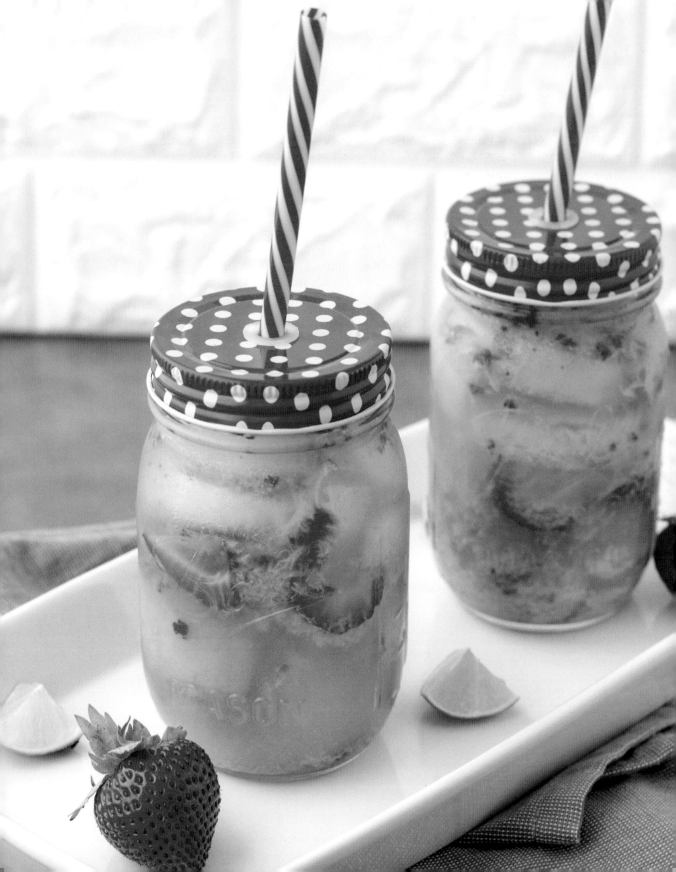

Mixed Berry Hard Lemonade

This is one of my favorite drinks to make when I am entertaining friends and family in the summer months. It is a light and refreshing crowd-pleaser. If you are hosting a backyard get-together, try quadrupling the recipe and making a pitcher to serve to your guests. Alternatively, you can set up a drinks bar with all the fixings and set out a recipe card. Not only does it make for a beautifully colorful setup, but it also gives your friends a chance to play bartender.

Makes 1 drink

2 ounces vodka

1½ ounces fresh lemon juice

⅓ ounce Low-Carb Simple Syrup (page 40)

2 ounces water

2 blackberries

2 blueberries

2 raspberries

1 strawberry, hulled and quartered

Lemon wheel, for garnish

1 Fill a cocktail shaker with ice. Add the vodka, lemon juice, simple syrup, water, blackberries, blueberries, raspberries, and strawberry. Cap and shake vigorously.

2 Pour the contents of the cocktail shaker into a pint-sized glass. Garnish with a lemon wheel.

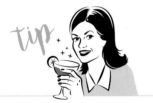

Try topping off this drink with club soda for an extra burst of fizzy refreshment.

CALORIES: 167 | FAT: 0 | PROTEIN: 1g | TOTAL CARBS: 8g | DIETARY FIBER: 2g | NET CARBS: 6g | ERYTHRITOL: 8g

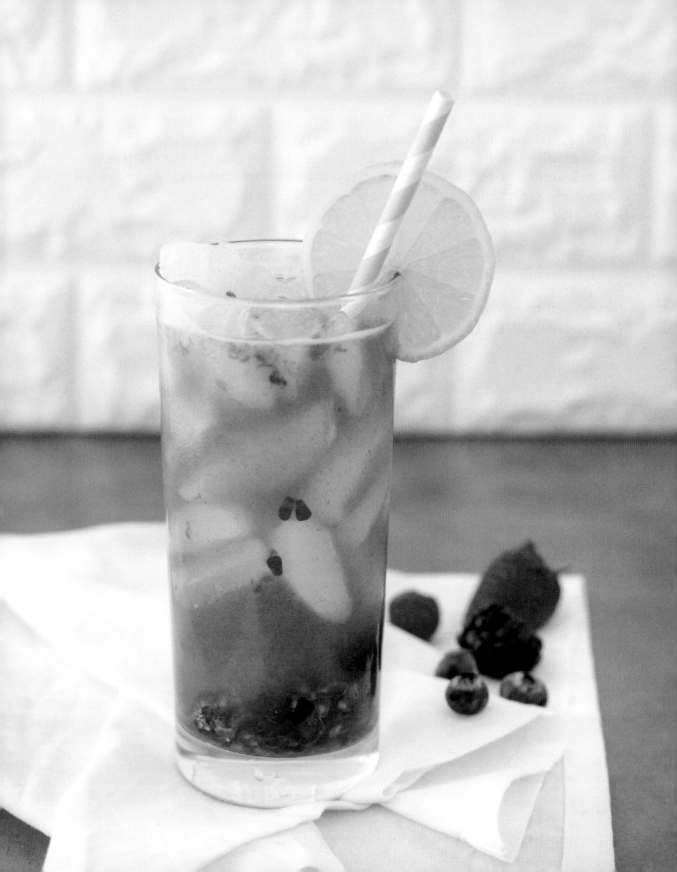

Kamikaze Shooter

A traditional Kamikaze shot is made with vodka, triple sec, and lime juice. Triple sec is a very sweet orange-flavored liqueur. It has more than 10 grams of carbohydrates per ounce. To get that traditional taste without adding unnecessary sugars, I use erythritol and pure orange extract instead. I think the end result could trick even the most refined drinking palates.

Makes 1 shot

FOR THE RIM OF THE GLASS (OPTIONAL):

1 teaspoon fresh lime juice

1 teaspoon coarse sea salt

FOR THE SHOT:

1½ ounces vodka

1 ounce fresh lime juice

¼ ounce Low-Carb Simple Syrup (page 40)

2 drops of pure orange extract

TO RIM THE GLASS (OPTIONAL):

1 Pour the lime juice onto a small plate.

2 Pour the salt onto a separate small plate.

3 Swirl the rim of a large shot glass in the lime juice, then swirl it in the salt to coat the rim.

TO MAKE THE SHOT:

1 Fill a cocktail shaker with ice. Add the vodka, lime juice, simple syrup, and orange extract. Cap and shake vigorously.

2 Strain the contents of the cocktail shaker into the salted shot glass or into a large shot glass.

CALORIES: 112 | FAT: 0 | PROTEIN: 0 | TOTAL CARBS: 2g | DIETARY FIBER: 0 | NET CARBS: 2g | ERYTHRITOL: 6g

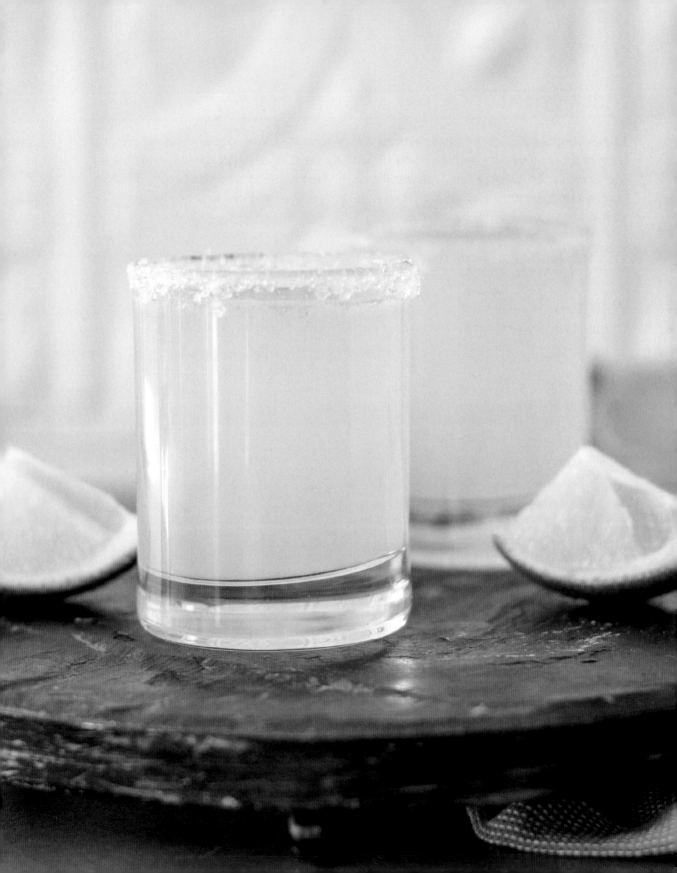

Bloody Mary

You've got to love a drink that doubles as a meal. Bloody Mary cocktails have almost become the kitschy knickknack of the drink world. There is a restaurant near me that serves their Bloody Marys with all the usual pickled vegetables and then takes it a step further by garnishing them with fried macaroni and cheese, chicken wings, a slider, and even a mini taco. I think I am just fine with a perfectly cooked strip of bacon and some briny pickled vegetables.

Makes 1 drink

2 ounces vodka

4 ounces Bloody Mary Mix (page 44)

1 celery stalk, for garnish

Olives, for garnish

1 strip crispy bacon, for garnish (optional)

Pickled vegetables, for garnish (optional)

1 Fill a cocktail shaker with ice. Add the vodka and Bloody Mary mix. Cap and shake vigorously.

2 Pour the contents of the shaker into a pint-sized glass. Garnish with celery, olives, bacon, and pickled vegetables, if desired, or any other fun keto foods you have on hand.

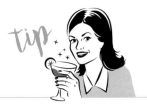

tip

For an extra flavor kick, try rimming the glass with celery salt. Delicious!

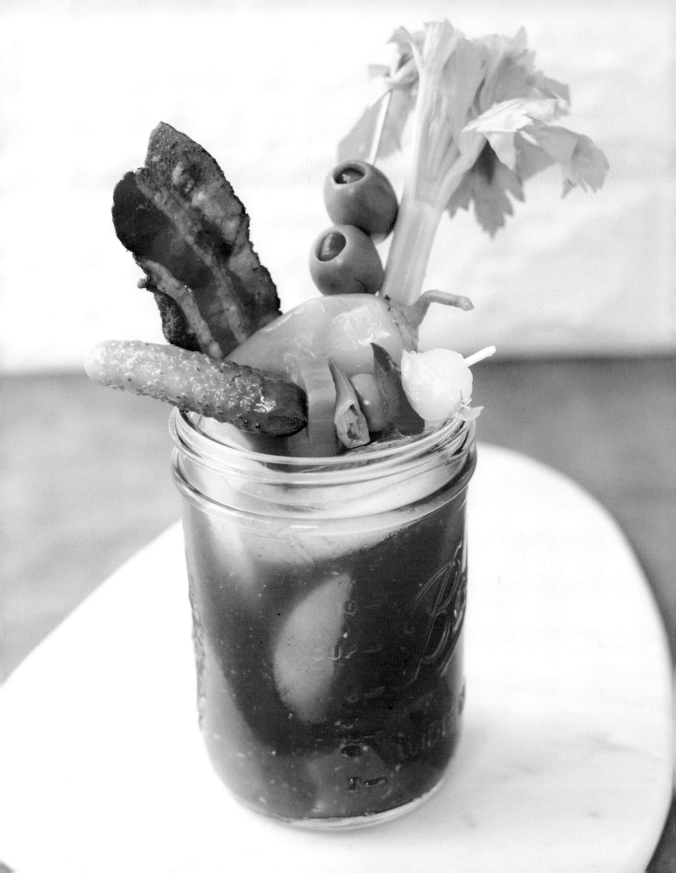

Moscow Mule

A traditional Moscow Mule is made with vodka, lime juice, and ginger beer. Ginger beer is typically very high in carbs, so as a work-around, I use my own ginger syrup, which is sweetened with erythritol, and then use club soda to get that perfect mule fizz.

Makes 1 drink

2 ounces vodka

1 ounce fresh lime juice

3 ounces Ginger Syrup (page 42)

Crushed ice

4 ounces club soda

Lime wheel, for garnish

Sprig of fresh mint, for garnish

1 Fill a cocktail shaker with ice. Add the vodka, lime juice, and ginger syrup. Cap and shake vigorously.

2 Fill a 16-ounce copper mug with crushed ice. Strain the contents of the cocktail shaker into the ice-filled mug and top with club soda.

3 Garnish with a lime wheel and a sprig of fresh mint.

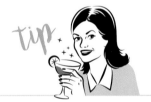

tip

This cocktail is also amazing as an Irish Mule when made with Irish whiskey.

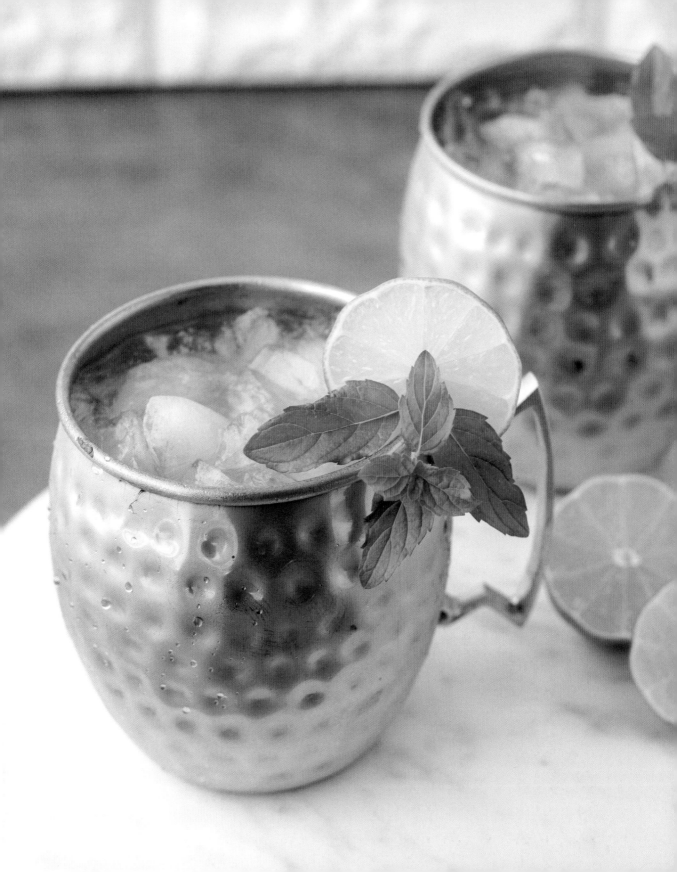

Salty Dog

Did you know that the only difference between a Greyhound and a Salty Dog is the salted rim? True story. Historically this drink was made with tequila, but on most menus these days, you will see it made with vodka instead.

Makes 1 drink

FOR THE RIM OF THE GLASS:

½ ounce fresh grapefruit juice

1 tablespoon coarse sea salt

FOR THE DRINK:

1½ ounces vodka

3 ounces fresh grapefruit juice

Grapefruit wedge, for garnish

TO RIM THE GLASS:

1 Pour the grapefruit juice onto a small plate.

2 Pour the salt onto a separate small plate.

3 Swirl the rim of a rocks glass in the grapefruit juice, then swirl it in the salt to coat the rim.

TO MAKE THE DRINK:

1 Fill a cocktail shaker three-quarters of the way full with ice. Add the vodka and grapefruit juice. Cap and shake vigorously.

2 Pour the contents of the cocktail shaker into the salted rocks glass.

3 Garnish with a grapefruit wedge.

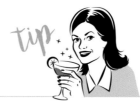

If you are buying grapefruit juice and not squeezing it fresh, be sure to look for a brand that is free of added sugars.

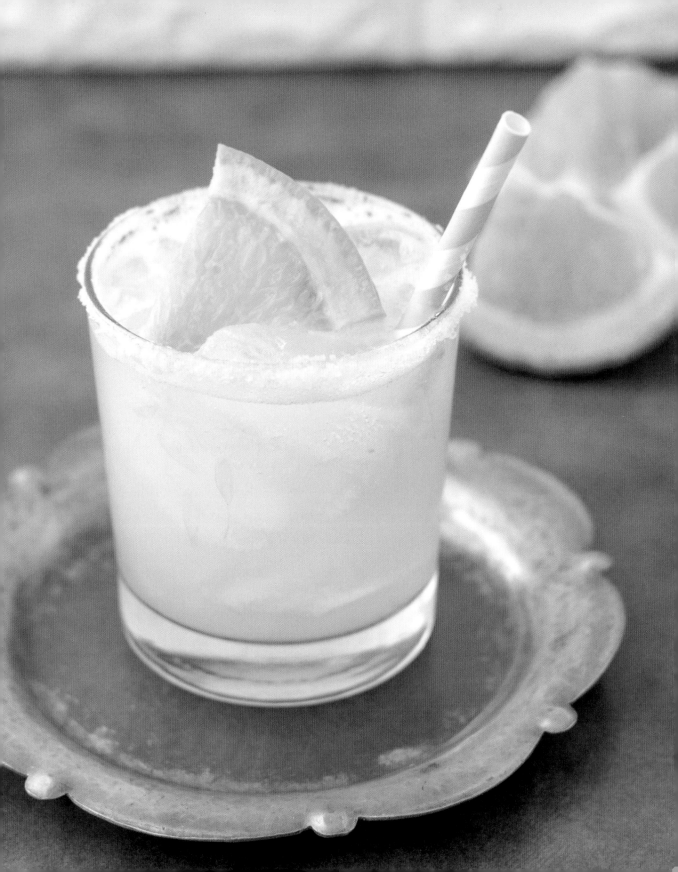

Strawberry-Basil Lemon Drop

If you are a fan of the classic Lemon Drop, then you will love this strawberry-basil variation. The basil in this drink adds a new depth of flavor and complements the sour citrus notes beautifully. The perfect drink for a low-carb girls' night!

Makes 1 drink

FOR THE RIM OF THE GLASS:

½ ounce fresh lemon juice

1 tablespoon granular erythritol

FOR THE DRINK:

3 large strawberries, divided

½ lemon, cut into wheels, divided

5 fresh basil leaves, cut into thin strips, plus more for garnish

1 ounce fresh lemon juice

½ ounce Low-Carb Simple Syrup (page 40)

1½ ounces vodka

TO RIM THE GLASS:

1   Pour the lemon juice onto a small plate.

2   Pour the erythritol onto a separate small plate.

3   Swirl the rim of a martini glass in the lemon juice, then swirl it in the erythritol to coat the rim.

TO MAKE THE DRINK:

1   Cut a slit in the bottom of one of the strawberries and one of the lemon wheels and place them on the rim of the martini glass as a garnish.

2   Remove the tops of the remaining 2 strawberries and slice.

3   Put the sliced strawberries, remaining lemon wheels, basil leaves, lemon juice, and simple syrup in a cocktail shaker. Muddle until the fruits are crushed and have released their juices.

4   Add the vodka to the cocktail shaker and fill with ice. Cap and shake vigorously.

5   Strain the mixture into the rimmed martini glass and garnish with basil.

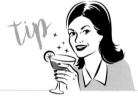

tip

For another fun fruit-and-herb fusion, try making this drink with blueberries and fresh rosemary.

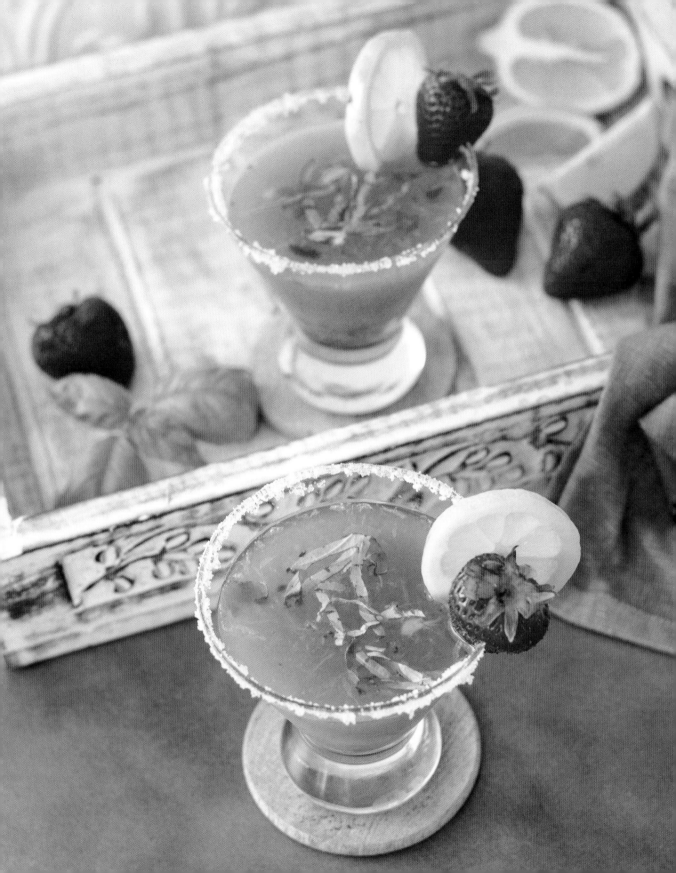

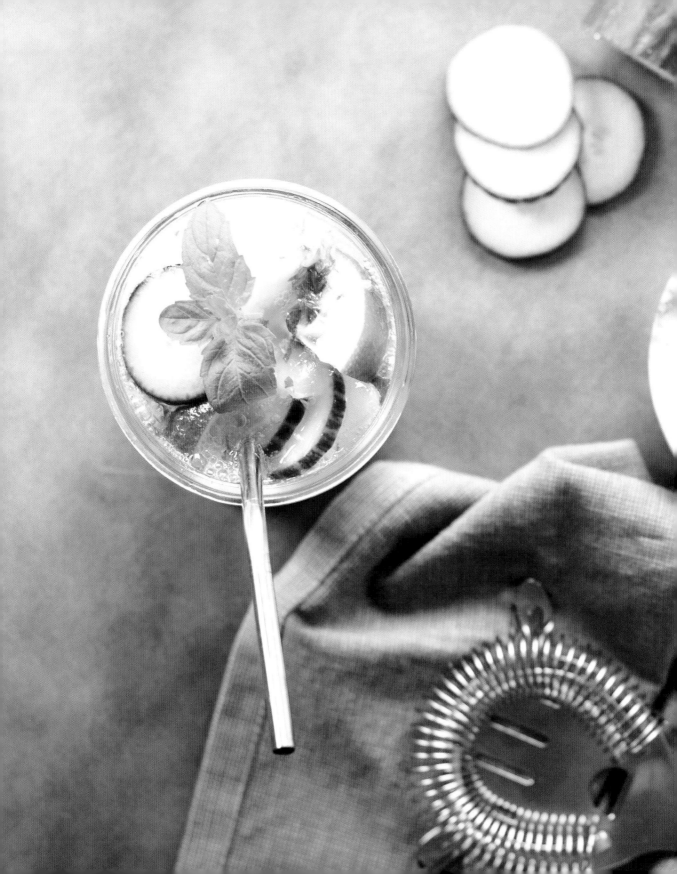

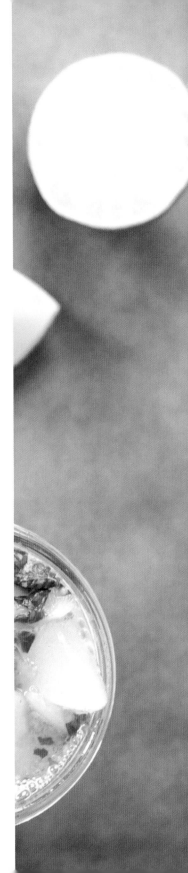

RUM
DRINKS

NET CARBS
4g

Blackberry Cobbler

All the flavors of a warm and comforting blackberry cobbler in a cool and refreshing beverage. This drink is also delicious with spiced rum.

Makes 1 drink

1½ ounces white rum

6 blackberries

¼ ounce Low-Carb Simple Syrup (page 40)

¼ teaspoon pure vanilla extract

Club soda

Sprig of fresh mint, for garnish (optional)

1 Combine the rum, blackberries, simple syrup, and vanilla extract in a cocktail shaker. Muddle until the berries are crushed and have released their liquid.

2 Fill a pint-sized glass with ice. Strain the contents of the cocktail shaker into the ice-filled glass and top with club soda.

3 Stir and garnish with a sprig of fresh mint, if desired.

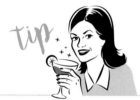

Try changing things up and making this drink with a mixture of blackberries, raspberries, and strawberries for a Mixed Berry Cobbler variation.

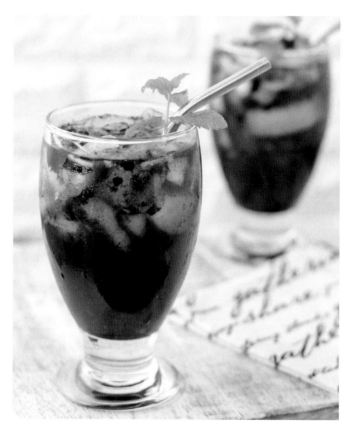

CALORIES: 110 | FAT: 0 | PROTEIN: 0 | TOTAL CARBS: 5g | DIETARY FIBER: 1g | NET CARBS: 4g | ERYTHRITOL: 6g

Dark 'n' Stormy

The Dark 'n' Stormy gets its name from the layering of colors used to make the drink: the "dark" part is rum, which is floated on top, and the "stormy" part is the ginger beer below it. As in the case of the Moscow Mule (page 64), I had to get a little creative with this one to get that amazing ginger beer flavor. The sweet-and-spicy nature of homemade ginger syrup and the fizziness of club soda are the perfect pairing for a drink that accurately represents the original.

Makes 1 drink

2 ounces Ginger Syrup (page 42)

1½ ounces fresh lime juice

4 ounces club soda

2 ounces dark rum

Lime wheel, for garnish

1   Fill a large rocks glass with ice. Pour the ginger syrup and lime juice over the ice and top with the club soda.

2   Stir gently to mix, but not so vigorously that the club soda goes flat. Top with the dark rum as a floater.

3   Garnish with a lime wheel.

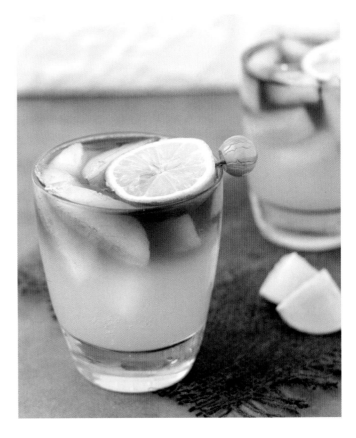

RUM
DRINKS

NET CARBS

5g

Cucumber Mojito

The cucumber in this mojito recipe adds an extra burst of freshness to an already refreshing drink. For an extra-fruity element, trying muddling in some fresh blueberries.

Makes 1 drink

5 thin slices English cucumber, plus more for garnish

8 fresh mint leaves, plus more for garnish

½ lime, cut into 4 wedges

½ ounce fresh lime juice

⅓ ounce Low-Carb Simple Syrup (page 40)

2 ounces white rum

5 ounces club soda

1   Fill a pint-sized glass with ice.

2   Put the cucumber, mint, lime wedges, lime juice, and simple syrup in a cocktail shaker. Muddle until the lime and cucumber are smashed and have released their juices.

3   Add the rum to the cocktail shaker. Cap and shake vigorously.

4   Pour the contents of the cocktail shaker into the ice-filled glass. Top with the club soda and stir gently.

5   Garnish with cucumber and fresh mint.

CALORIES: 158 | FAT: 0 | PROTEIN: 2g | TOTAL CARBS: 7g | DIETARY FIBER: 2g | NET CARBS: 5g | ERYTHRITOL: 9g

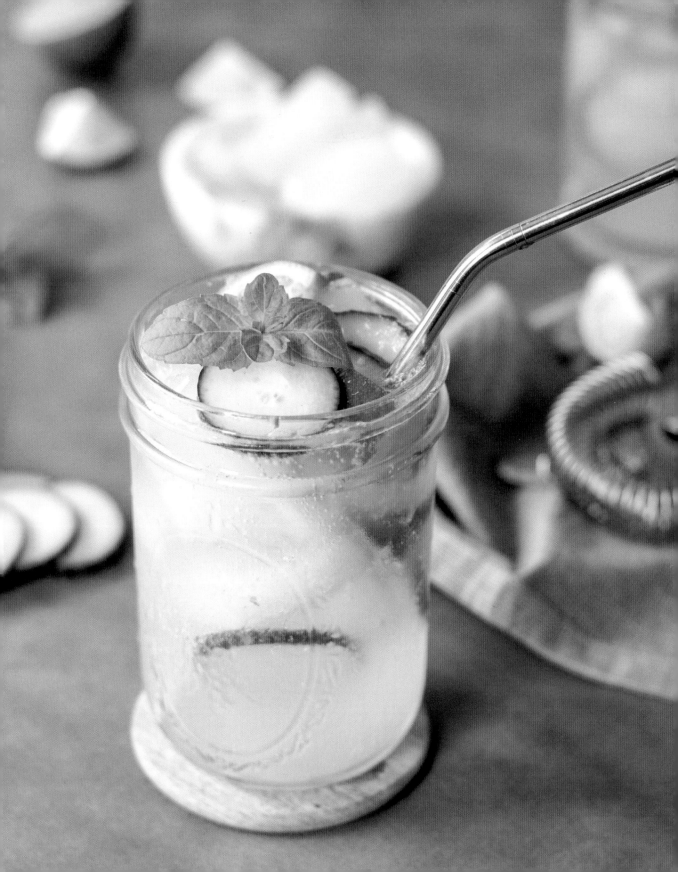

RUM
DRINKS

Frosted Rum Cake

All the delicious flavors of a frosted cake in delicious drink form. It's like the flavors of fall have met a tropical island right in your glass.

Makes 1 drink

FOR THE RIM OF THE GLASS:

2 tablespoons raw almonds

1 tablespoon granular erythritol

½ ounce water

FOR THE DRINK:

½ teaspoon pure vanilla extract

¼ teaspoon pure almond extract

¼ teaspoon pure orange extract

1½ teaspoons powdered erythritol

2 ounces spiced rum

1 cup ice

¼ cup coconut milk

¼ cup heavy cream

Orange slice, for garnish (optional)

TO RIM THE GLASS:

1 Combine the almonds and granular erythritol in a high-powered blender or food processor. Pulse until well combined and finely ground.

2 Pour the water onto a small plate.

3 Pour the almond and sweetener mixture onto a separate small plate.

4 Swirl the rim of a pint-sized glass in the water, then swirl it in the almond and sweetener mixture to coat the rim.

TO MAKE THE DRINK:

1 Combine the extracts, powdered erythritol, rum, ice, coconut milk, and cream in a blender. Blend until smooth and creamy. Pour the mixture into the rimmed glass.

2 Garnish with an orange slice, if desired.

CALORIES: 356 | FAT: 25g | PROTEIN: 2g | TOTAL CARBS: 3g | DIETARY FIBER: 1g | NET CARBS: 2g | ERYTHRITOL: 18g

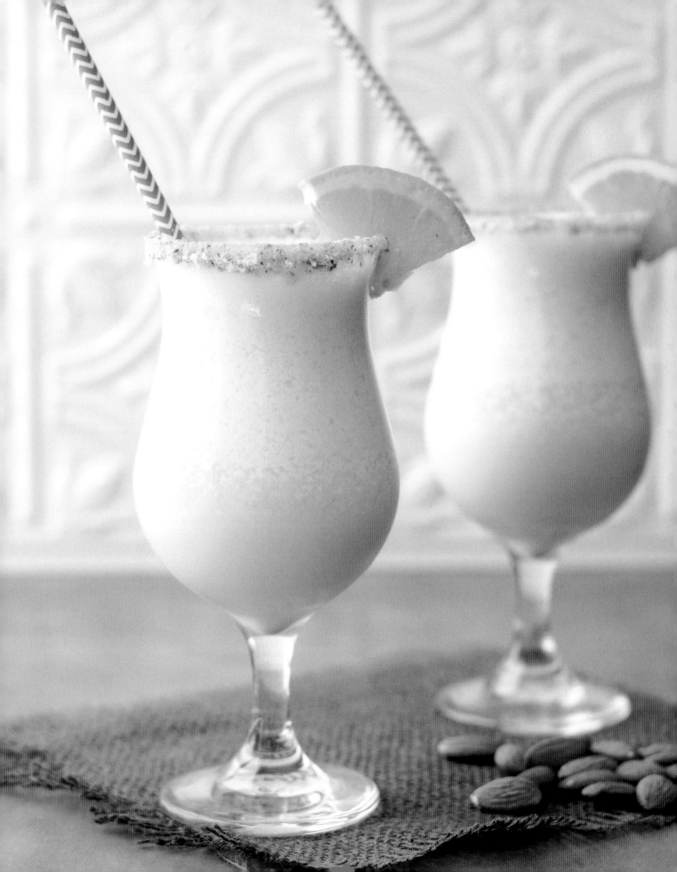

Piña Colada

Want to be instantly whisked away to white sandy beaches, crashing waves, and all the other amazing sights and sounds of the tropics? Yeah, me too! Well, for now, just kick off your shoes, pour yourself a low-carb Piña Colada, let the sunshine hit your face, and pretend.

Makes 1 drink

1 cup ice

½ cup coconut cream (see note)

1½ ounces white rum

1 ounce Low-Carb Simple Syrup (page 40)

½ ounce fresh lime juice

1 teaspoon pure pineapple extract

Fresh cherry, for garnish (optional)

Slice of fresh pineapple, for garnish (optional)

1   Combine all the ingredients in a blender and pulse until smooth and creamy.

2   Pour the contents of the blender into a hurricane glass. Garnish with a cherry and a pineapple slice, if desired.

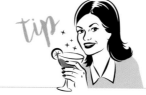

tip

To make this into a Lava Flow, puree a handful of fresh strawberries and pour them into the glass before pouring in the Piña Colada mixture. Then watch the lava rise!

note

Be sure not to confuse coconut cream with cream of coconut. Coconut cream is very thick and unsweetened, and coconut is the sole ingredient. It is most commonly found canned. Cream of coconut, on the other hand, is a thick liquid that is very sweet.

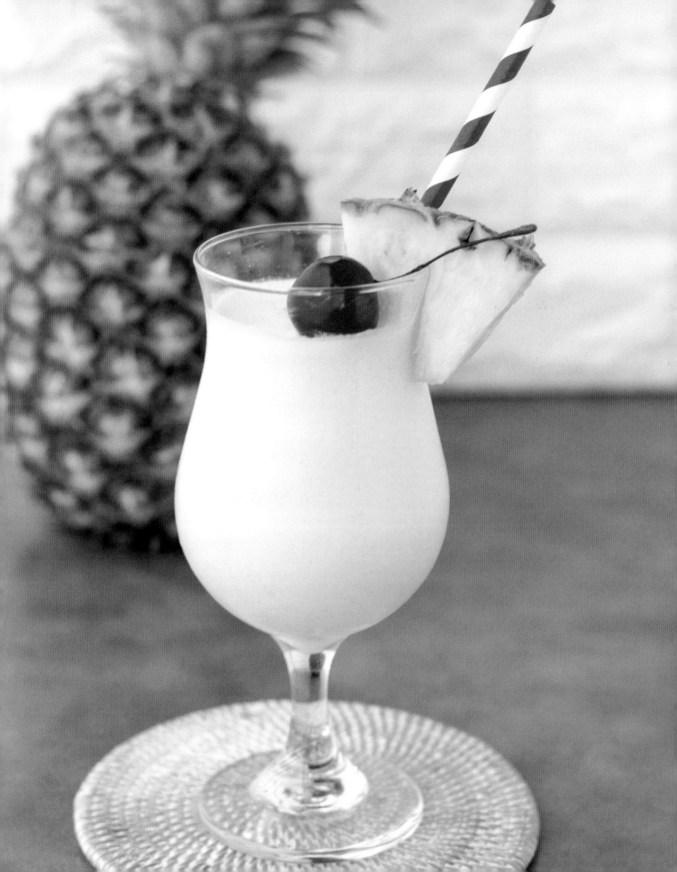

Raspberry Flip

Before you take a look at this recipe and run away screaming, let me tell you a little bit about the history of the flip. The name dates back to a time when hot pokers were used to "flip" a drink—to make it boil and froth. Over time, an egg white was added to produce the froth, and the drink ceased to be served hot. While the flip is not a common drink on today's modern craft cocktail menus, it is definitely worth revisiting. I have no doubt that you will be pleasantly surprised and will soon be flipping out with all your friends.

Makes 1 drink

1½ ounces white rum

½ ounce fresh lemon juice

½ ounce Low-Carb Simple Syrup (page 40)

10 raspberries, plus more for garnish

1 egg white

1 Combine all the ingredients in a blender and pulse until smooth and frothy.

2 Fill a cocktail shaker with ice. Pour the mixture from the blender into the shaker. Cap and shake vigorously.

3 Strain the contents of the cocktail shaker into a 12-ounce glass and garnish with raspberries.

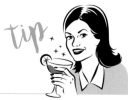

tip

If you are hesitant to use the egg white, try making this drink with a splash of heavy cream instead.

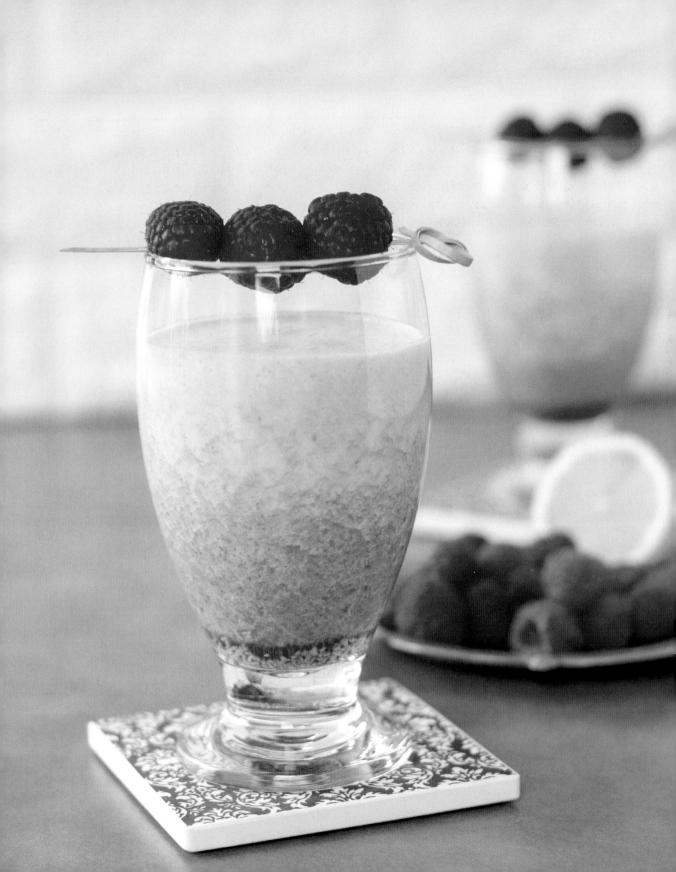

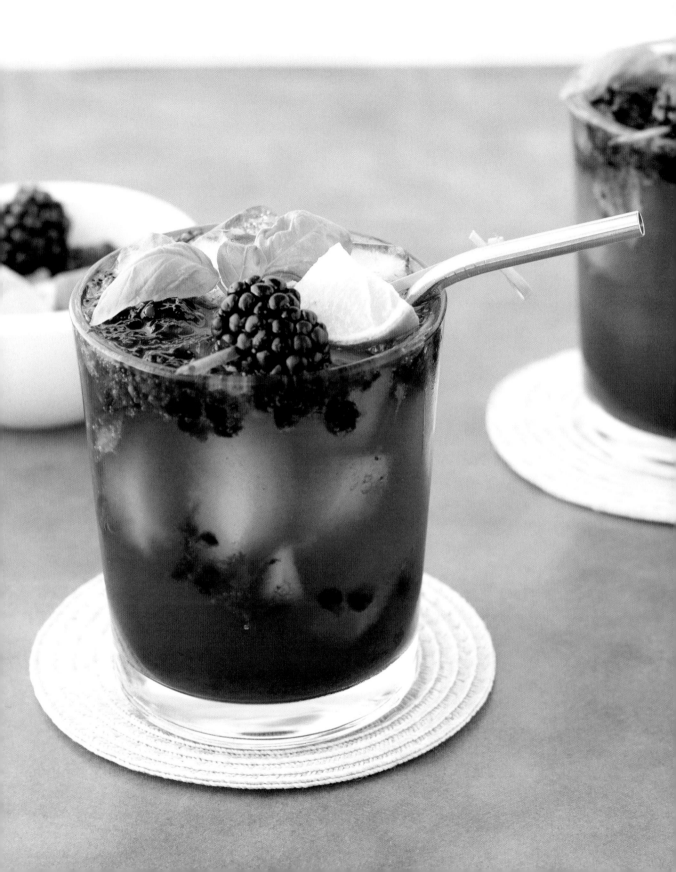

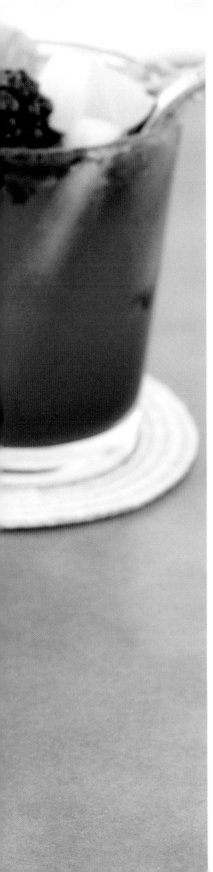

GIN
drinks

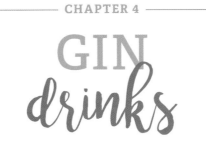

Blackberry-Basil Gin Fizz

The origin of the Gin Fizz can be traced back to one of my favorite cities in the world, New Orleans. In 1888, bar owner Henry C. Ramos invented the Ramos Gin Fizz at his bar on Gravier Street, the Imperial Cabinet Saloon. In the traditional version, there is a frothed egg white, much like in the Raspberry Flip on page 80, but in more modern versions, the egg is usually omitted, as it is in this recipe.

Makes 1 drink

2 ounces dry gin

1 ounce fresh lime juice

¼ ounce Low-Carb Simple Syrup (page 40)

4 blackberries, plus more for garnish

2 fresh basil leaves, plus more for garnish

Club soda

Lime wedge, for garnish

1   Fill a rocks glass with ice.

2   Combine the gin, lime juice, simple syrup, blackberries, and basil in a cocktail shaker. Muddle until the fruit is crushed and has released its juices.

3   Pour the contents of the cocktail shaker into the ice-filled glass. Top with club soda.

4   Garnish with a lime wedge, blackberries, and basil.

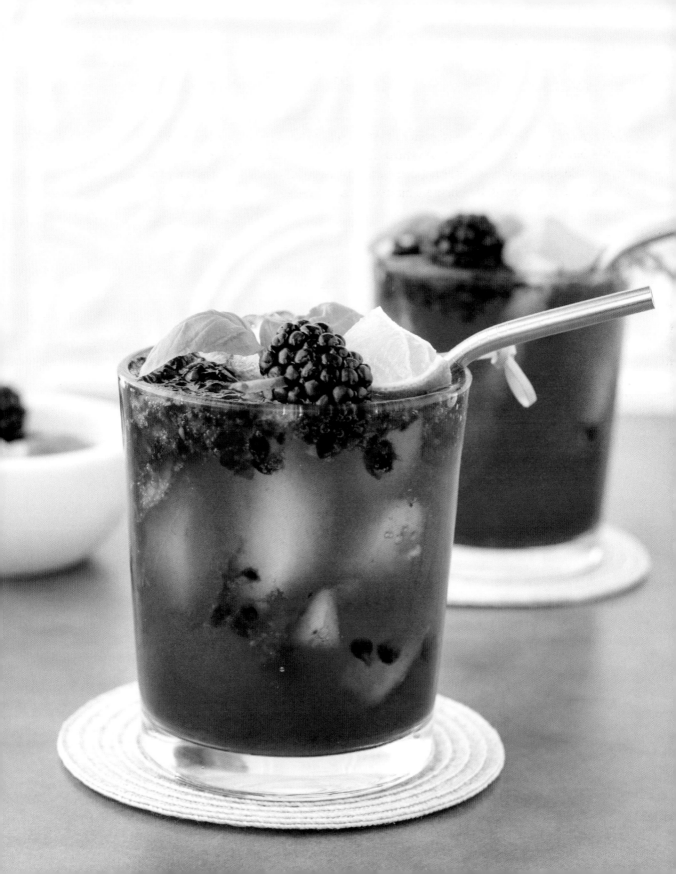

Dirty Gibson

A classic Gibson contains gin, dry vermouth, and cocktail onions. What makes this Gibson dirty? Well, as naughty as the term may sound, it refers only to the addition of cocktail onion brine. As explained in the "Bartending Lingo" guide on pages 12 and 13, what makes a martini dirty is the addition of some of the juice from the drink's garnish. In a classic dirty martini, olive juice is added, but for this Dirty Gibson, I've added cocktail onion brine.

Makes 1 drink

2 ounces dry gin

½ ounce dry vermouth

½ ounce cocktail onion brine

2 cocktail onions, for garnish

1   Fill a cocktail shaker with ice. Add the gin, vermouth, and onion brine. Cap and shake vigorously, until the shaker is very cold and frost starts to form on the outside.

2   Strain the contents of the cocktail shaker into a chilled martini glass and garnish with the cocktail onions.

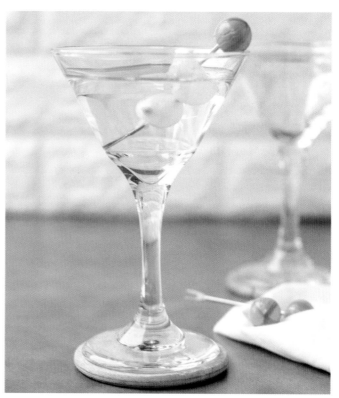

Gin Rickey

The Gin Rickey dates back to the 1880s in Washington, D.C. Its invention is most commonly credited to Missouri-born lobbyist Colonel Joe Rickey, who was nicknamed the "Alcoholic Forefather." While I'm not sure I would want the word alcoholic *in any of my nicknames, it would be pretty cool to have a drink named after me that would still be popular centuries later.*

Makes 1 drink

2 ounces dry gin

1 ounce fresh lime juice

4 ounces club soda

Lime wheel or wedge, for garnish

1 Fill a large rocks glass with ice.

2 Pour the gin and lime juice over the ice. Top with the club soda and stir.

3 Garnish with a lime wheel or wedge.

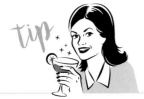

This drink is also delicious made with whiskey.

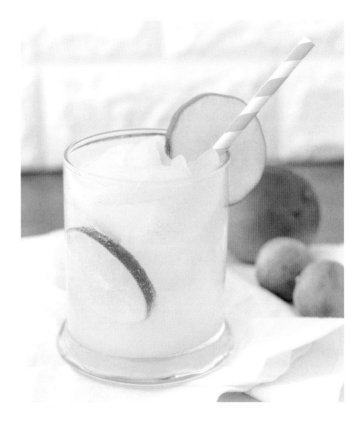

Grapefruit Dreamin'

The name "Grapefruit Dreamin'" is so appropriate for this drink because I have been dreaming about it ever since I first made it. The fresh tarragon in this recipe really adds something special that, to be honest, even I wasn't expecting. This flavor combination threw some extra fuel on the fire for my love of fruit-and-herb fusions.

Makes 1 drink

2 ounces dry gin

2 ounces fresh grapefruit juice

⅓ ounce Low-Carb Simple Syrup (page 40)

2 sprigs of fresh tarragon, divided

2 ounces sparkling wine

Grapefruit wedge, for garnish (optional)

1 Fill a cocktail shaker with ice. Add the gin, grapefruit juice, simple syrup, and one of the tarragon sprigs. Cap and shake vigorously.

2 Fill a large rocks glass with ice. Strain the contents of the cocktail shaker into the ice-filled glass. Top with the sparkling wine.

3 Garnish with a grapefruit wedge, if using, and the remaining sprig of tarragon.

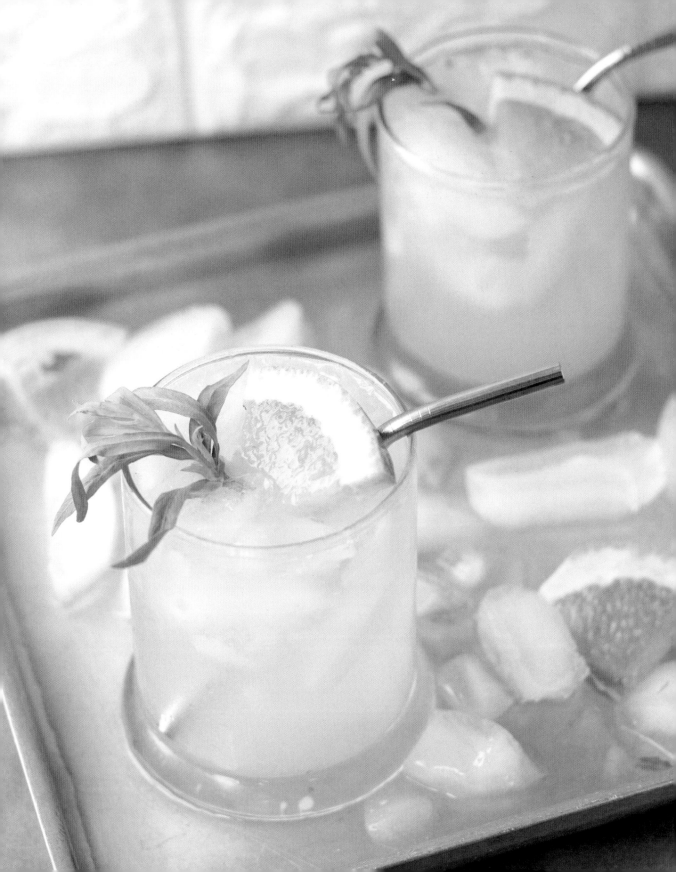

Lavender Ginny

I have to admit something to you. When I first started writing this book, I wasn't sure I was a fan of gin. I thought that writing the gin section would be a tricky task to tackle. But as I developed these recipes, I found that I actually quite enjoy the taste of gin. There is so much more to gin than boring old gin and tonics.

Makes 1 drink

1½ ounces dry gin

1 ounce fresh lime juice

1 tablespoon dried lavender buds, plus more for garnish

¼ ounce Low-Carb Simple Syrup (page 40)

Club soda

Lime wedge, for garnish

1 Fill a large rocks glass with ice.

2 Fill a cocktail shaker with ice. Add the gin, lime juice, lavender buds, and simple syrup. Cap and shake vigorously.

3 Strain the contents of the cocktail shaker into the ice-filled glass. Top with club soda.

4 Garnish with a lime wedge and lavender buds.

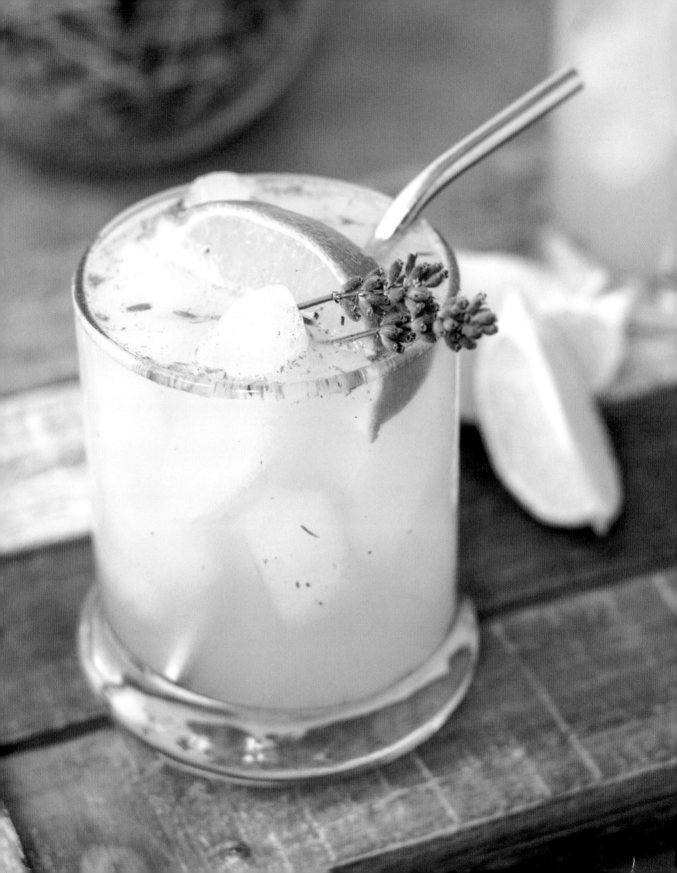

NET CARBS
4g

Lemon-Basil Crush

If you haven't tasted the amazingly refreshing flavor combination that is lemon and basil, prepare to have your taste buds blown. Combining various fruits and herbs quickly became a passion as I set out to write this book. They work together so harmoniously to create intense, bright flavor.

Makes 1 drink

3 fresh basil leaves

1 ounce fresh lemon juice

¼ ounce Low-Carb Simple Syrup (page 40)

3 lemon wedges

1½ ounces dry gin

Club soda

Lemon wheel, for garnish

Basil crown, for garnish

1 Combine the basil leaves, lemon juice, simple syrup, and lemon wedges in a cocktail shaker. Muddle until the lemons and basil are crushed and have released their juices.

2 Add the gin to the cocktail shaker. Cap and shake vigorously.

3 Fill a large rocks glass with ice. Strain the contents of the cocktail shaker into the ice-filled glass. Top with club soda.

4 Garnish with a lemon wheel and a basil crown.

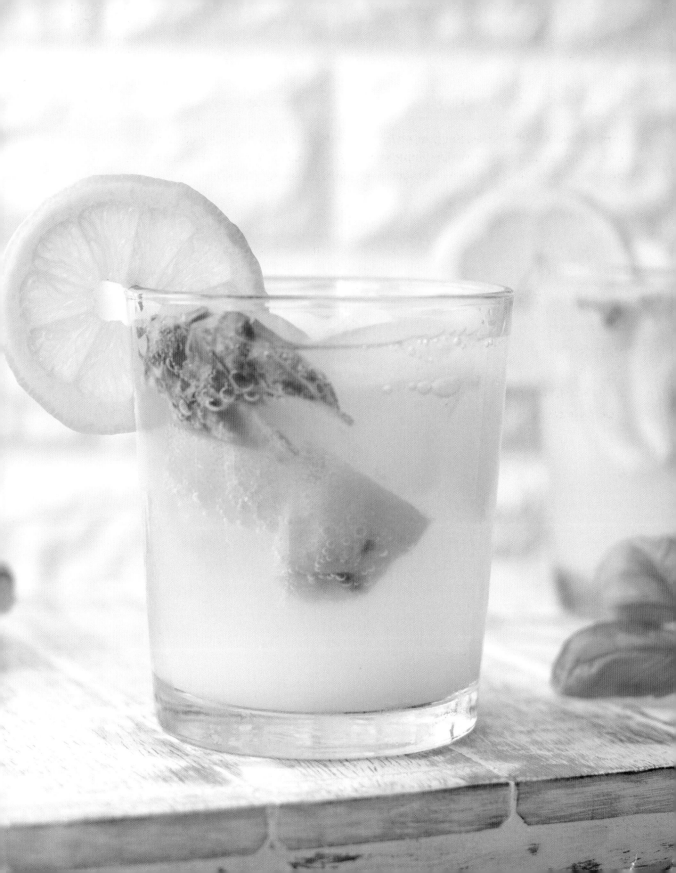

Tom Collins

The very first edition of the classic Bartender's Guide *by Jerry Thomas was published in 1862. Thomas was known as the father of American mixology. It is said that the Tom Collins recipe in the 1887 edition of his book is the first one ever recorded. In his version, the type of alcohol being used was specified after the drink name—for example, "Tom Collins Gin" or "Tom Collins Whiskey." It was those who came after him who deemed the Tom Collins a gin drink.*

Makes 1 drink

1½ ounces dry gin

1 ounce fresh lemon juice

½ ounce Low-Carb Simple Syrup (page 40)

Club soda

Lemon wedge, for garnish

1 Combine the gin, lemon juice, and simple syrup in a Collins glass and stir.

2 Fill the glass with ice and top with club soda.

3 Garnish with a lemon wedge.

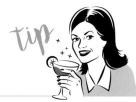

tip

There are many ways to enjoy a Collins. Try these other delicious variations and choose your favorite. Simply swap out the liquor and you are good to go. Collins drinks go by a variety of men's names, but here are some of the versions I've seen floating around: John Collins (whiskey), Juan Collins (tequila), Ron Collins (rum), and Vodka Collins, which, strangely enough, seems to go by that moniker alone. I vote that we name it Tim Collins, Tom's younger, more popular brother.

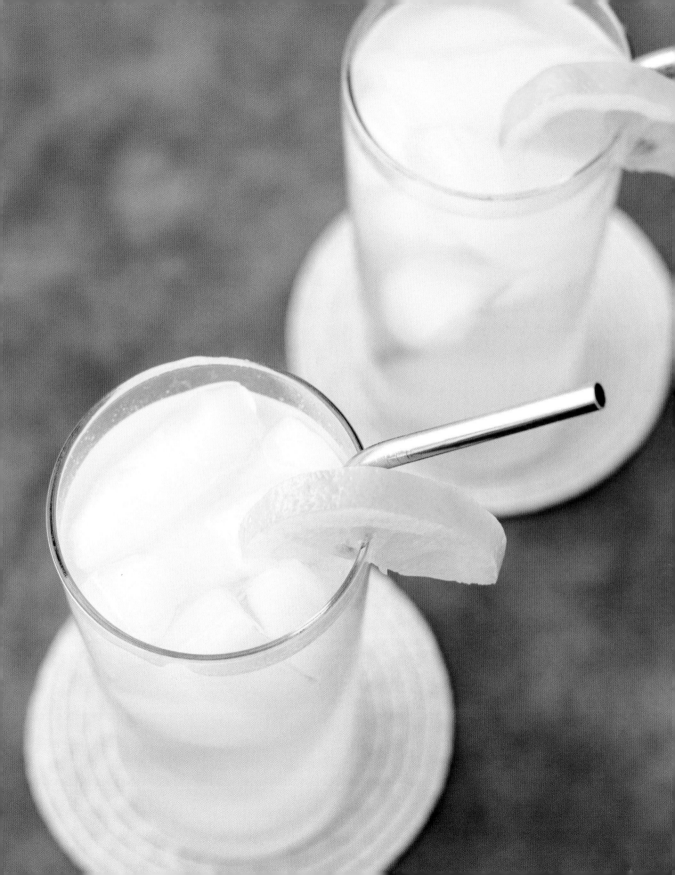

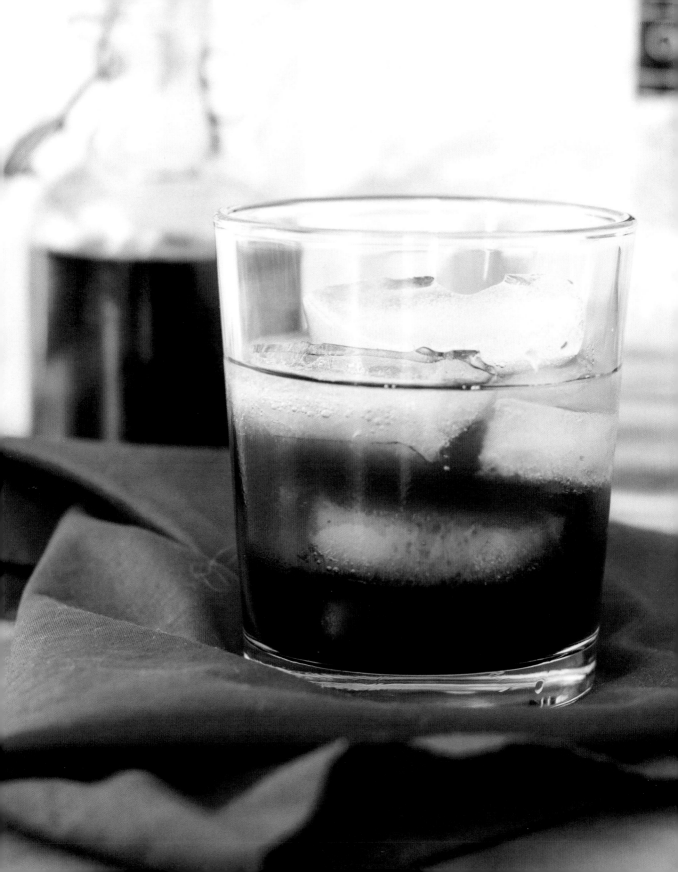

TEQUILA *drinks*

Bloody Maria

If there are two drinks that make day drinking seem socially acceptable, they are the Bloody Mary and the mimosa. These two are the stars of weekend brunch menus everywhere. In fact, a good Bloody Mary usually comes so loaded up with food garnishes that it almost makes a meal all on its own. Well, the Bloody Mary has a Mexican sister, and her name is Bloody Maria. This traditional tomato juice–based cocktail kicks things up a notch by substituting tequila for the vodka in the original.

Makes 1 drink

FOR THE RIM OF THE GLASS:

½ ounce fresh lime juice

1 tablespoon celery salt

FOR THE DRINK:

2 ounces silver tequila

4 ounces Bloody Mary Mix (page 44)

Assortment of fresh and pickled vegetables, for garnish

TO RIM THE GLASS:

1 Pour the lime juice onto a small plate.

2 Pour the celery salt onto a separate small plate.

3 Swirl the rim of a pint-sized glass in the lime juice, then swirl the glass in the celery salt to coat the rim.

TO MAKE THE DRINK:

1 Fill the rimmed glass with ice. Add the tequila and Bloody Mary mix and stir to combine.

2 Garnish with the fresh and pickled vegetables of your choice.

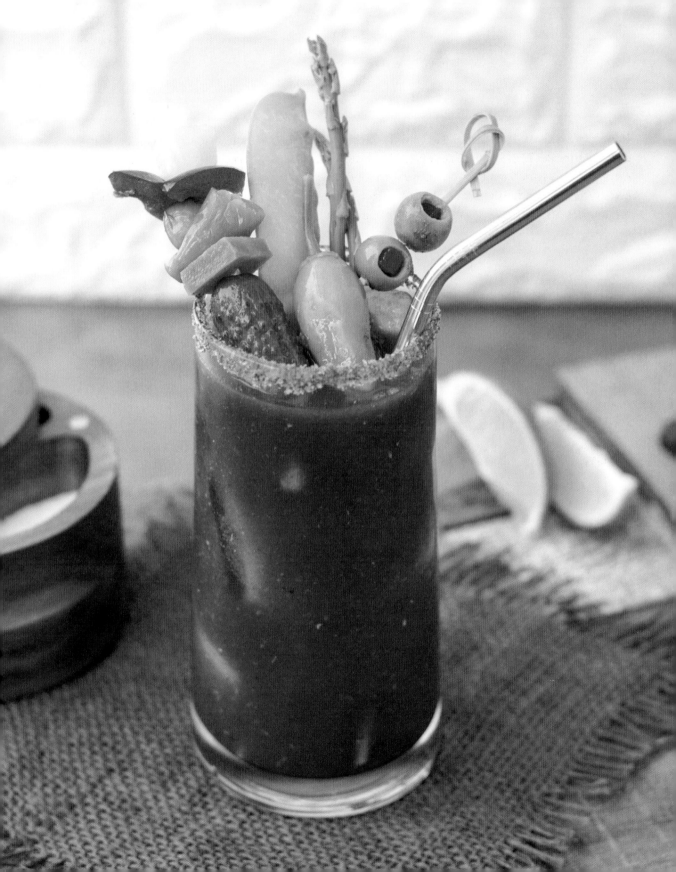

Cucumber-Jalapeño Margarita

I love the spiciness of jalapeños paired with the cooling vibe of cucumbers. Throw some citrus into the mix and you have a match made in heaven.

Makes 1 drink

FOR THE RIM OF THE GLASS:

½ ounce fresh lime juice

1 tablespoon coarse sea salt

FOR THE DRINK:

2 ounces silver tequila

2 ounces Sweet-and-Sour Mix (page 46)

2 slices English cucumber

2 slices jalapeño pepper

2 drops of pure orange extract

2 ounces club soda

TO RIM THE GLASS:

1 Pour the lime juice onto a small plate.

2 Pour the salt onto a separate small plate.

3 Swirl the rim of a 12-ounce glass in the lime juice, then swirl it in the salt to coat the rim.

TO MAKE THE DRINK:

1 Fill a cocktail shaker with ice. Add the tequila, sweet-and-sour mix, cucumber, jalapeño, and orange extract. Cap and shake vigorously.

2 Pour the contents of the cocktail shaker into the rimmed glass and top with the club soda.

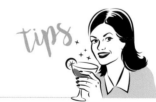

tips

For a deeper jalapeño-and-cucumber-infused flavor, mix together the tequila, sweet-and-sour mix, cucumber, jalapeño, and orange extract and refrigerate for 3 to 4 hours before serving.

If spicy isn't your thing, try making this drink with a handful of mixed berries for a light and fruity version.

CALORIES: 147 | FAT: 0.1g | PROTEIN: 0.2g | TOTAL CARBS: 3.3g | DIETARY FIBER: 0.2g | NET CARBS: 3.1g | ERYTHRITOL: 12g

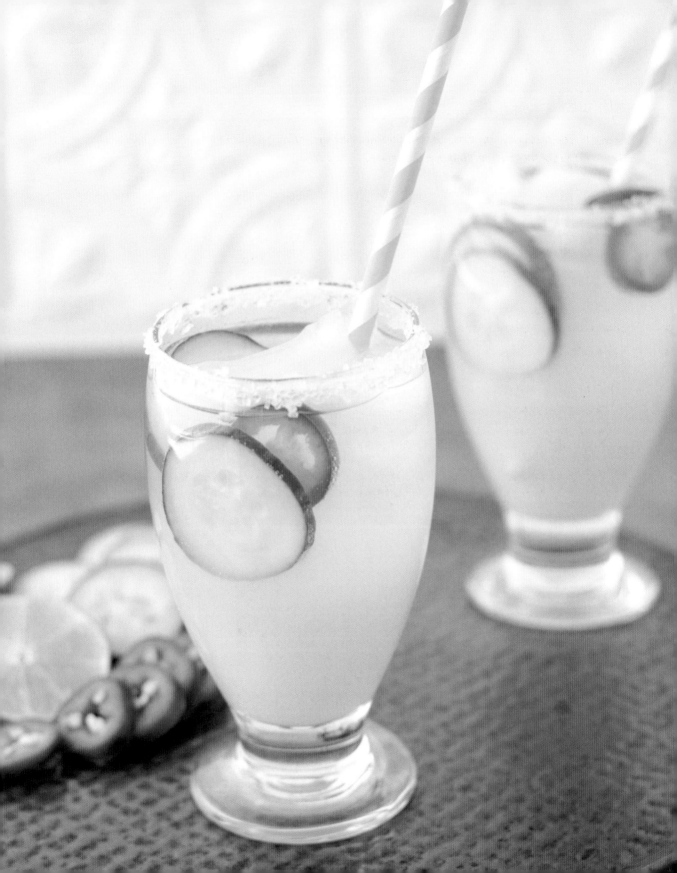

Mama's Margarita

Take your Taco Tuesday to the next level with a thirst-quenching margarita.

Makes 1 drink

FOR THE RIM OF THE GLASS:

½ ounce fresh lime juice

1 teaspoon coarse sea salt

FOR THE DRINK:

½ lime, cut into wedges

2 ounces silver tequila

2 ounces Sweet-and-Sour Mix
(page 46)

2 drops of pure orange extract

Lime wheel, for garnish

TO RIM THE GLASS:

1 Pour the lime juice onto a small plate.

2 Pour the salt onto a separate small plate.

3 Swirl the rim of a margarita glass in the lime juice, then swirl it in the salt to coat the rim.

TO MAKE THE DRINK:

1 Fill a cocktail shaker with ice. Squeeze the lime wedges over the ice, then drop the wedges into the shaker. Add the tequila, sweet-and-sour mix, and orange extract. Cap and shake vigorously.

2 Strain the contents of the cocktail shaker into the rimmed margarita glass.

3 Garnish with a lime wheel.

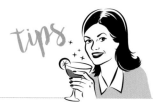

tips.

For a strawberry margarita, puree a few strawberries and add them to the cocktail shaker before shaking.

If you prefer a frozen margarita, pour the contents of the cocktail shaker (minus the lime wedges) into a blender and pulse until smooth.

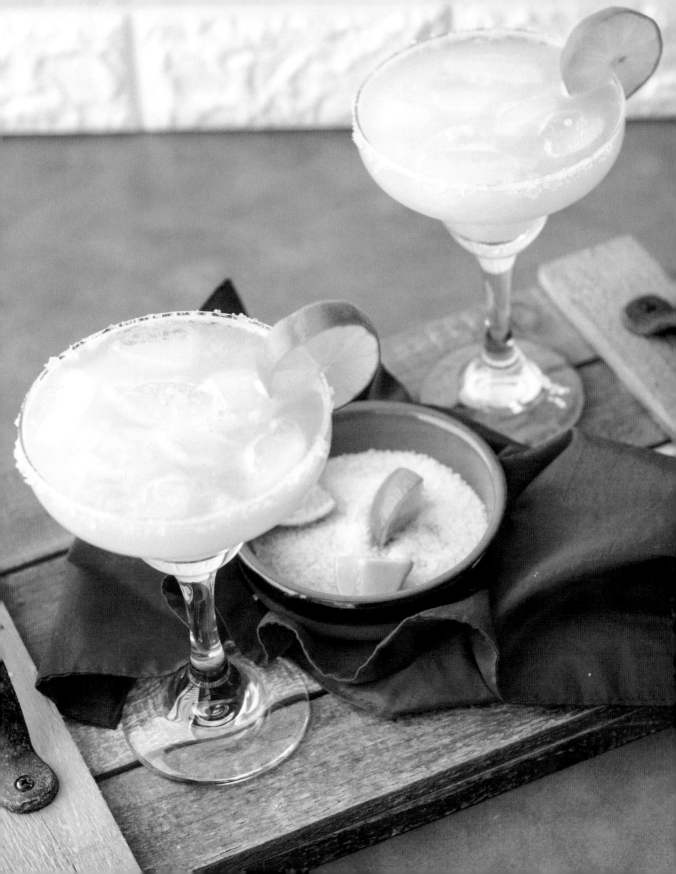

Pretty-in-Pink Paloma

In Mexico, a traditional Paloma is made with tequila, fresh lime juice, and some sort of sweet grapefruit-flavored soda, like Jarritos. In the United States, it's often made with a fruit-flavored soda like Fresca or Squirt. For this low-carb version, I opted to skip both the sugary and the artificially sweetened soda options and sweeten the drink with the natural sweetener erythritol, freshly squeezed grapefruit juice, and club soda. Now that I think of it, that sounds like a refreshing combination all on its own, even without the tequila.

Makes 1 drink

FOR THE RIM OF THE GLASS:

½ ounce fresh pink or ruby red grapefruit juice

1 tablespoon coarse sea salt

FOR THE DRINK:

1½ ounces silver tequila

2 ounces fresh pink or ruby red grapefruit juice

½ ounce fresh lime juice

¼ ounce Low-Carb Simple Syrup (page 40)

Club soda

Pink or ruby red grapefruit wedge, for garnish

TO RIM THE GLASS:

1 Pour the grapefruit juice onto a small plate.

2 Pour the salt onto a separate small plate.

3 Swirl the rim of a Collins glass in the grapefruit juice, then swirl it in the salt to coat the rim.

TO MAKE THE DRINK:

1 Fill the rimmed glass with ice.

2 Fill a cocktail shaker with ice. Add the tequila, grapefruit juice, lime juice, and simple syrup. Cap and shake vigorously.

3 Strain the contents of the cocktail shaker into the ice-filled glass. Top with club soda.

4 Garnish with a grapefruit wedge.

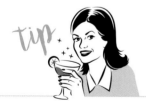

tip

If you are not a fan of tequila, try making this drink with white rum or even vodka. If making it with rum or vodka, I recommend rimming the glass with granular erythritol instead of coarse sea salt.

CALORIES: 131 | FAT: 0 | PROTEIN: 0 | TOTAL CARBS: 7g | DIETARY FIBER: 0 | NET CARBS: 7g | ERYTHRITOL: 6g

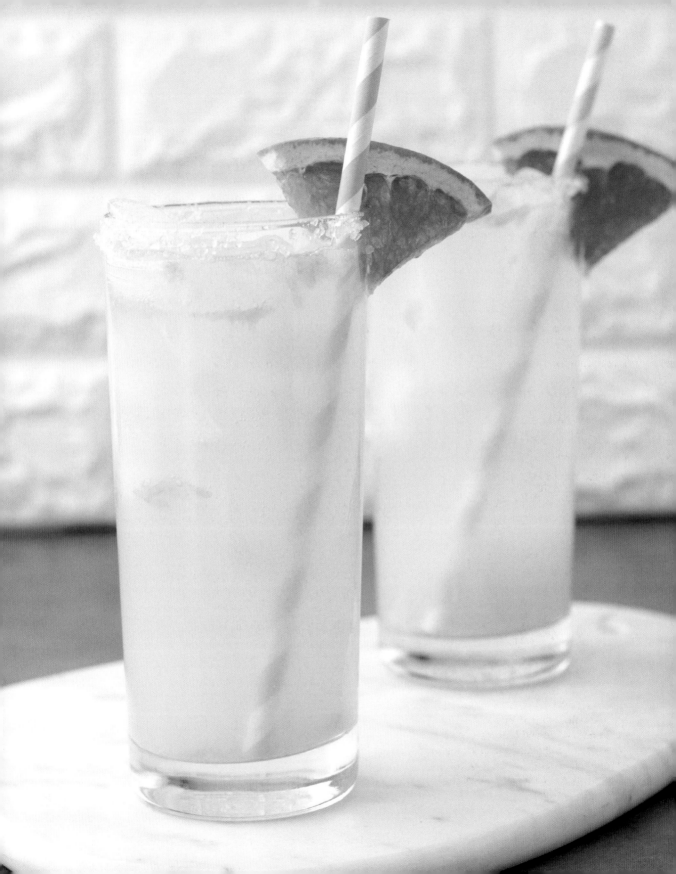

Rosemary-Lime Tequila Spritzer

This drink is so light and refreshing, perfect for a hot summer's day. If you're entertaining friends, quadruple the recipe to make a pitcher. It's the perfect way to perk up your party routine.

Makes 1 drink

Leaves from 1 sprig of fresh rosemary

1½ ounces silver tequila

2 ounces fresh lime juice

¼ ounce Low-Carb Simple Syrup (page 40)

Pinch of fine sea salt

Club soda

Lime wedge, for garnish (optional)

Sprig of fresh rosemary, for garnish (optional)

1 Fill a cocktail shaker with ice. Add the rosemary leaves, tequila, lime juice, simple syrup, and salt. Cap and shake vigorously.

2 Pour the contents of the cocktail shaker into a pint-sized glass. Top with club soda.

3 Garnish with a lime wedge and rosemary sprig, if desired.

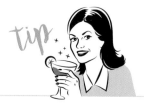

tip

Not a fan of tequila? Try making this drink with vodka or gin.

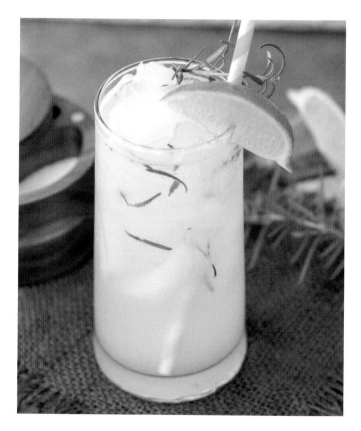

CALORIES: 119 | FAT: 0 | PROTEIN: 0 | TOTAL CARBS: 5g | DIETARY FIBER: 0 | NET CARBS: 5g | ERYTHRITOL: 6g

Brave Bull

You've probably heard of a White Russian, and you've likely even heard of a Black Russian, but have you heard of a Brave Bull? It's a tequila-fied Black Russian. Many drinks that are rooted in vodka history turn up with a tequila counterpart. Much like the Vodka Collins turned into the Juan Collins and the Bloody Mary (page 62) morphed into the Bloody Maria (page 98), the Brave Bull ditches vodka for the kicked-up flavor of tequila. While coffee liqueur and tequila might sound like a strange pairing, I think you will be pleasantly surprised.

Makes 1 drink

2 ounces silver tequila

1 ounce Homemade Coffee Liqueur (page 166)

Fill a rocks glass with ice. Add the tequila and coffee liqueur and stir to combine.

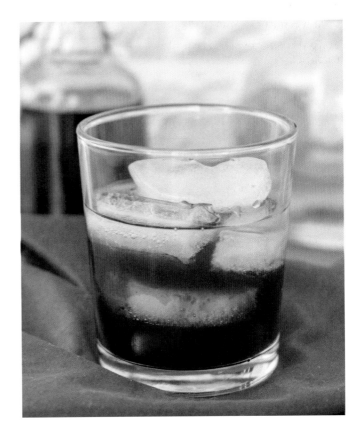

Strawberry Margarita Gummy Worms

This adult version of a childhood favorite really packs a punch—sweet, boozy, and silly all at once.

Makes 24 gummies (4 per serving)

10 hulled strawberries, fresh or frozen

2 ounces silver tequila

3 tablespoons grass-fed gelatin collagen protein

2 tablespoons powdered erythritol

1½ ounces fresh lime juice

SPECIAL EQUIPMENT:

Standard-sized silicone gummy worm mold with 24 wells

1 Combine the strawberries and tequila in a blender and pulse until smooth.

2 Pour the strawberry-and-tequila mixture into a medium saucepan and set over low heat. Add the gelatin, erythritol, and lime juice and whisk to dissolve the gelatin and combine the ingredients. Continue to heat for about 10 minutes, whisking frequently, until the mixture becomes pourable. It will start out very thick but will become thinner and smoother as it heats.

3 Transfer the mixture to a measuring cup or a bowl with a pour spout.

4 Quickly pour the mixture into the gummy worm mold and transfer to the refrigerator.

5 Refrigerate for 10 to 15 minutes, until set. Pop the gummy worms out of the mold and enjoy! Store leftovers in the refrigerator for up to a week.

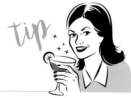

tip

Not a fan of tequila? Try making these gummy worms with rum or vodka.

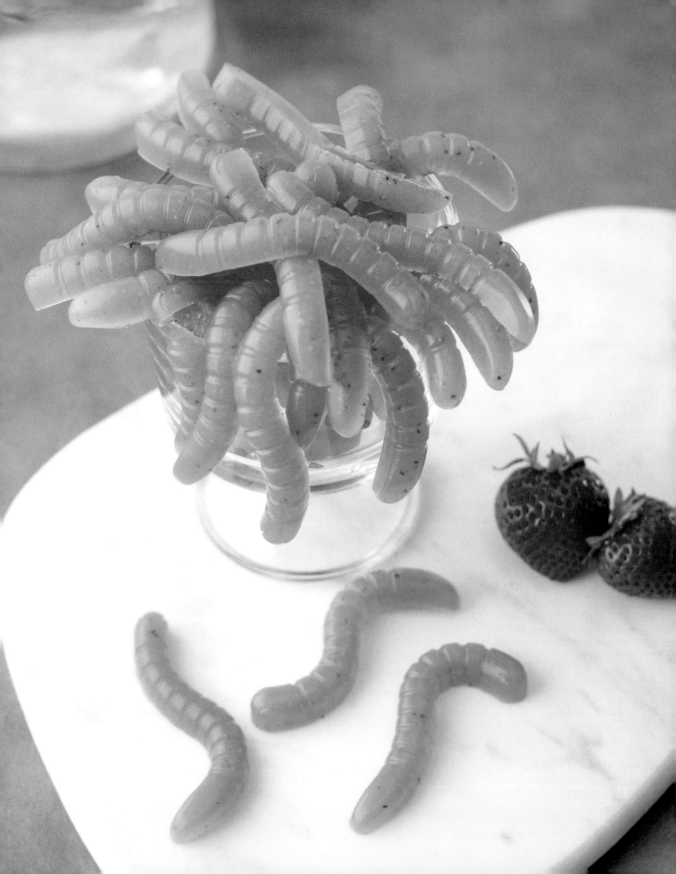

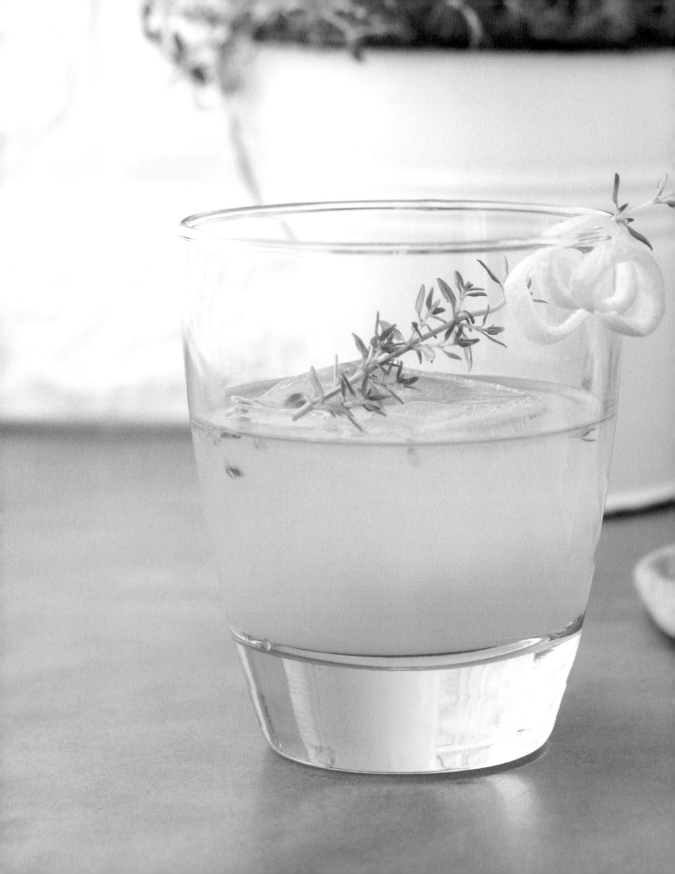

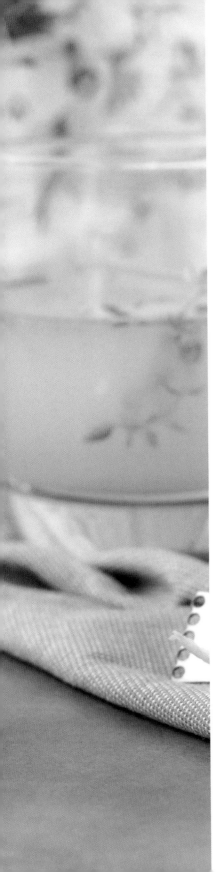
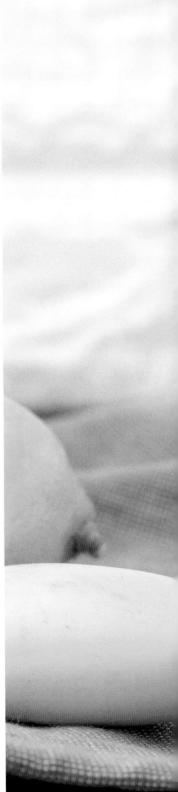

WHISKEY *drinks*

Irish Cold Brew

Who says your favorite morning beverage can't also be a part of your favorite cocktail? There are plenty of hot coffee cocktails, so I thought I would give cold brew its time to shine in the cocktail spotlight. Whiskey and coffee are always a great match. For a hot coffee drink made with whiskey, try my recipe for Irish Coffee (page 162).

Makes 1 drink

2 ounces Irish whiskey

6 ounces cold-brew coffee

2 ounces heavy cream

1 teaspoon powdered erythritol
(optional)

Fill a pint-sized glass with ice. Add the whiskey, coffee, and cream. Stir to combine. Stir in the erythritol, if using.

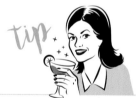

This is also amazing as a blended drink. Simply pour the finished drink into a blender and pulse until smooth. To make it extra creamy, add a few tablespoons of Fresh Whipped Cream (page 47) to the blender along with the drink.

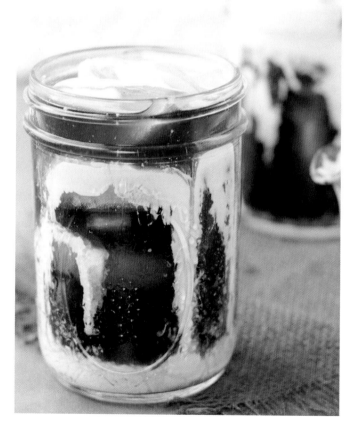

Whiskey Sour

A traditional Whiskey Sour has nearly 20 grams of carbs, and it all comes from sugar, making it a less-than-stellar option for those of us living a low-carb lifestyle. However, with my low-carbified version, you can once again indulge in this timeless classic.

Makes 1 drink _____

2 ounces whiskey

3 ounces Sweet-and-Sour Mix (page 46)

Fresh cherry, for garnish

Lime wedge, for garnish

1   Fill a large rocks glass with ice. Pour the whiskey over the ice and top with the sweet-and-sour mix.

2   Garnish with a cherry and a lime wedge.

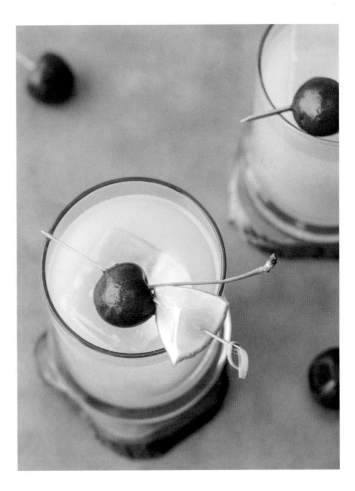

It's Whiskey Thyme

I love a good play on words almost as much as I love the flavors of whiskey and thyme together. This drink has one foot in spring and one foot in fall, making it perfect for almost any season.

Makes 1 drink

2 ounces whiskey

1 ounce Ginger Syrup (page 42)

½ ounce fresh lemon juice

2 sprigs of fresh thyme, divided

Lemon twist, for garnish

1 Fill a large rocks glass with ice.

2 Fill a cocktail shaker with ice. Add the whiskey, ginger syrup, lemon juice, and one of the thyme sprigs. Cap and shake vigorously.

3 Strain the contents of the cocktail shaker into the ice-filled rocks glass.

4 Garnish with the remaining thyme sprig and a lemon twist.

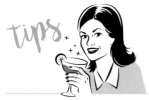

To make this drink extra refreshing, try topping it off with a little club soda.

For maximum flavor, infuse the thyme in the ginger syrup overnight.

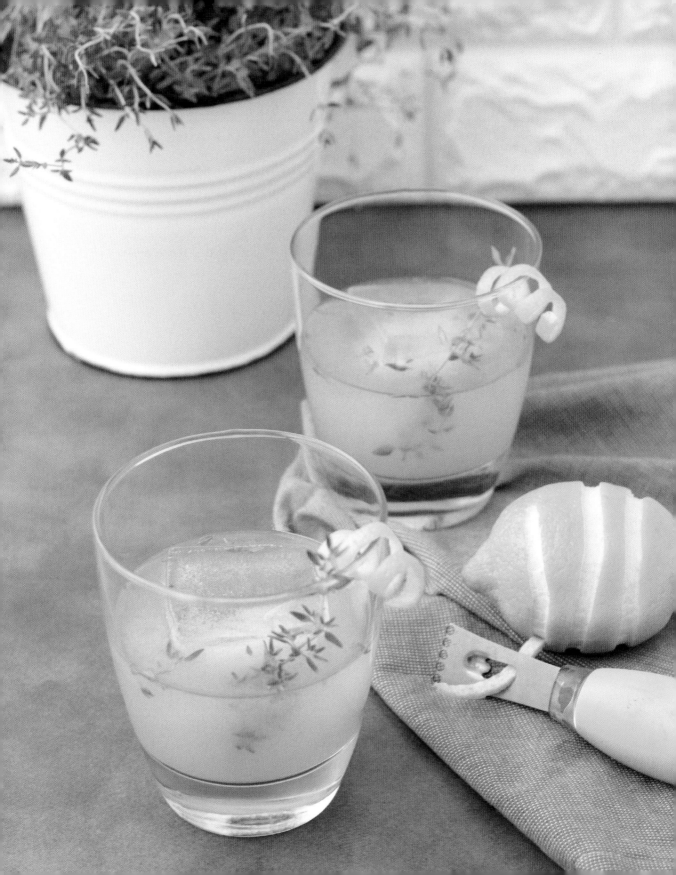

Manhattan

While attempting to trace the origin of the Manhattan, I was led down a path that diverged into wild stories, outlandish lore, and even a few seemingly dull moments in history. All the stories varied widely, but the one common denominator was that this drink did in fact originate in the borough of Manhattan, sometime in the late 1800s. While a Manhattan is traditionally made with whiskey, you can now find several variations: A Rob Roy is made with scotch. A Dry Manhattan is made with dry vermouth in place of sweet vermouth. A Cuban Manhattan is made with dark rum in place of whiskey. And a Tijuana Manhattan is made with añejo tequila. Because I prefer my Manhattan with a hint of orange flavor, I like to garnish it with a fresh orange twist, and occasionally I even use orange bitters in place of the angostura bitters.

Makes 1 drink

2 ounces whiskey

1 ounce sweet vermouth

2 dashes angostura bitters

Fresh cherry, for garnish

Orange twist, for garnish (optional)

1　Fill a cocktail shaker with ice. Add the whiskey, vermouth, and bitters. Stir until well chilled, about 20 seconds.

2　Strain the contents of the cocktail shaker into a chilled martini glass. Garnish with a cherry and an orange twist, if using.

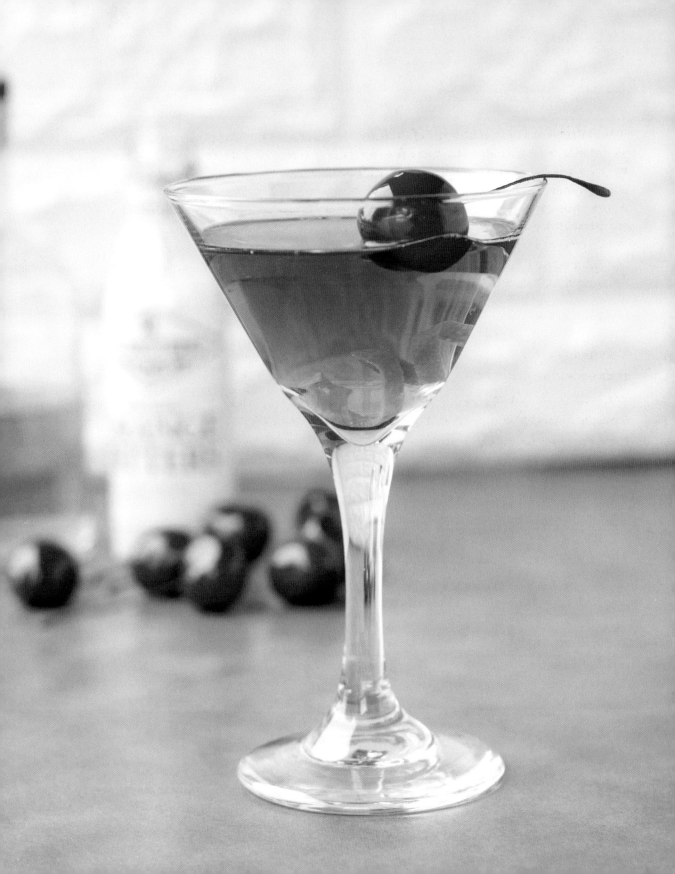

Mint Julep

The Mint Julep originated in the southern United States around the end of the eighteenth century, but it didn't reach iconic status until 1938, when it started being promoted by Churchill Downs Racetrack for the Kentucky Derby. Each year, more than a hundred thousand Mint Juleps are served during the two-day period of the Derby. So men, don your fedoras and bowler hats, and ladies, grab the biggest, floppiest, most ornate hat you can find, and mix yourself up a julep!

Makes 1 drink

Leaves from 4 sprigs of fresh mint, plus 1 sprig for garnish

½ ounce Low-Carb Simple Syrup (page 40)

2½ ounces whiskey

Crushed ice

1 Put the mint leaves and simple syrup in a 12-ounce glass. Muddle well to release the natural oils from the mint.

2 Add the whiskey to the glass and fill it with crushed ice. Stir until well chilled, about 20 seconds.

3 Garnish with a sprig of fresh mint.

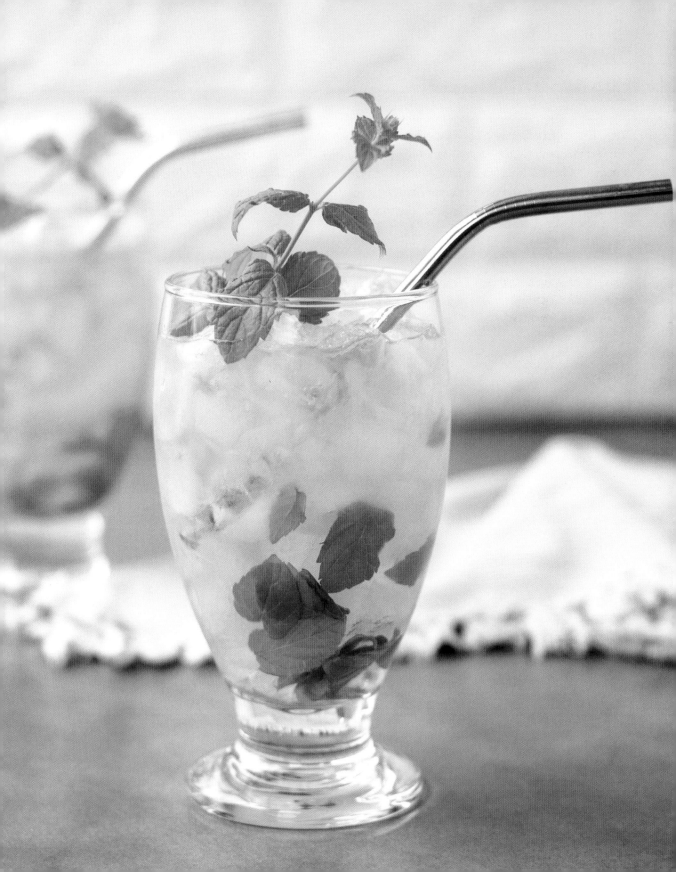

Old-Fashioned

The Old-Fashioned is about as old-fashioned as a cocktail can get. Like most classic cocktails, it can be traced back to the 1800s and is still alive and well today. Through the decades, and now even the centuries, the Old-Fashioned has hinted at refinement and culture while being approachable and timeless. Much like the Cosmopolitan (page 52) had a revival due to Sex and the City, *the Old-Fashioned saw a serious uptick when the dashing Don Draper of* Mad Men *was rarely seen without one in his hands.*

Makes 1 drink

1 teaspoon Low-Carb Simple Syrup (page 40)

1 teaspoon water

2 dashes of angostura bitters

2 orange wheels, divided

2 ounces whiskey

Fresh cherry, for garnish

Orange twist, for garnish (optional)

1 Put the simple syrup, water, bitters, and one of the orange wheels in a large rocks glass and muddle well to release the juice and aromatic oils from the orange. Discard the crushed orange wheel.

2 Fill the glass with ice, add the whiskey, and stir until well chilled, about 20 seconds.

3 Garnish with a cherry, an orange twist (if using), and the remaining orange wheel.

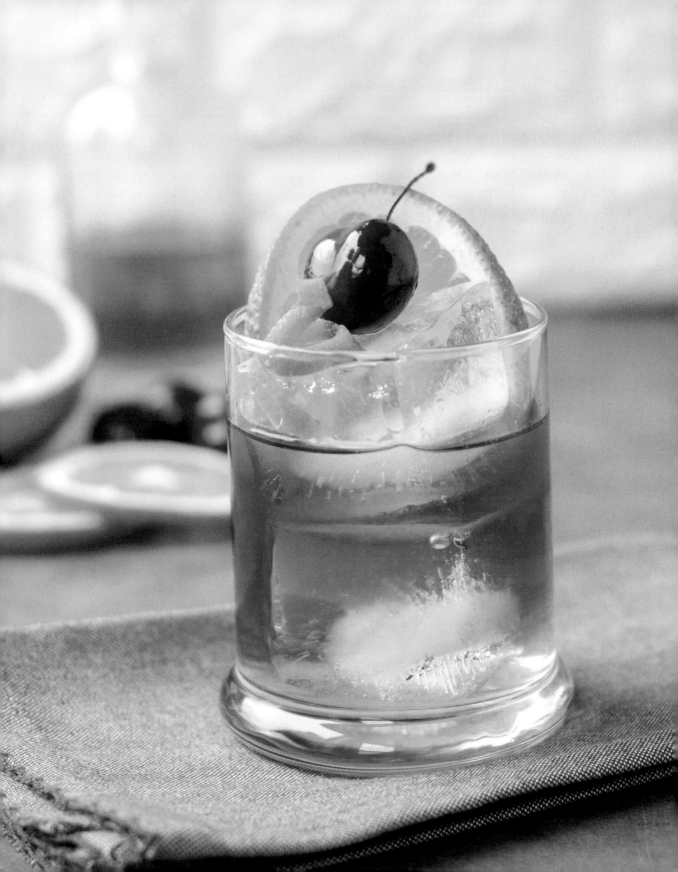

Pickleback

If there was ever going to be a "hair of the dog" drink, the Pickleback is it. Science is calling out brine as a hangover cure. Well, it says that the acetic acid in the vinegar is an antidiuretic that contains electrolytes and absorbs salt. Looks like you've got yourself the perfect breakfast drink. Be sure to check out pages 35 to 37 for more creative hangover hacks.

Makes 1 drink

1½ ounces whiskey

1½ ounces pickle juice

1 Pour the whiskey into a chilled shot glass.

2 Pour the pickle juice into a separate chilled shot glass.

3 Shoot the whiskey, then drink the pickle juice as a chaser.

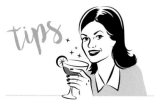

For a spicy spin on this unconventional shooter, try using the brine from pepperoncini or pickled jalapeños in place of the pickle juice.

To maximize the health benefits of pickle brine, I recommend buying a fermented pickle brand, such as Bubbies.

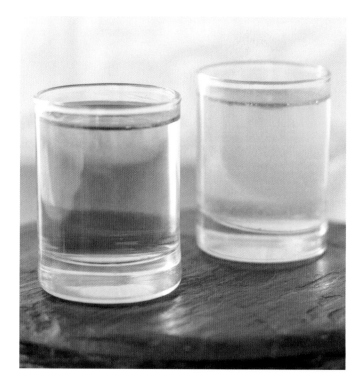

Rosemary's Baby

If you were to search for the term "Rosemary's Baby Cocktail" online, you would find that no two drinks contain the same set of ingredients. Of course, I had to throw my hat in the ring and make my own rendition. The bright freshness of lemon juice paired with woodsy rosemary is one of my favorite fruit-and-herb fusions.

Makes 1 drink

1½ ounces whiskey

1 ounce fresh lemon juice

⅓ ounce Low-Carb Simple Syrup (page 40)

2 sprigs of fresh rosemary, divided

Club soda

Lemon wedge, for garnish

1 Fill a large rocks glass with ice.

2 Fill a cocktail shaker with ice. Add the whiskey, lemon juice, simple syrup, and the leaves from one of the rosemary sprigs. Cap and shake vigorously.

3 Strain the contents of the cocktail shaker into the ice-filled glass and top with club soda.

4 Garnish with the remaining sprig of rosemary and a lemon wedge.

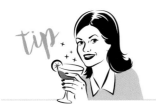

Not a fan of whiskey? This drink is also fantastic made with vodka!

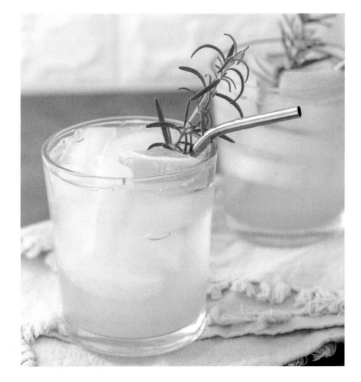

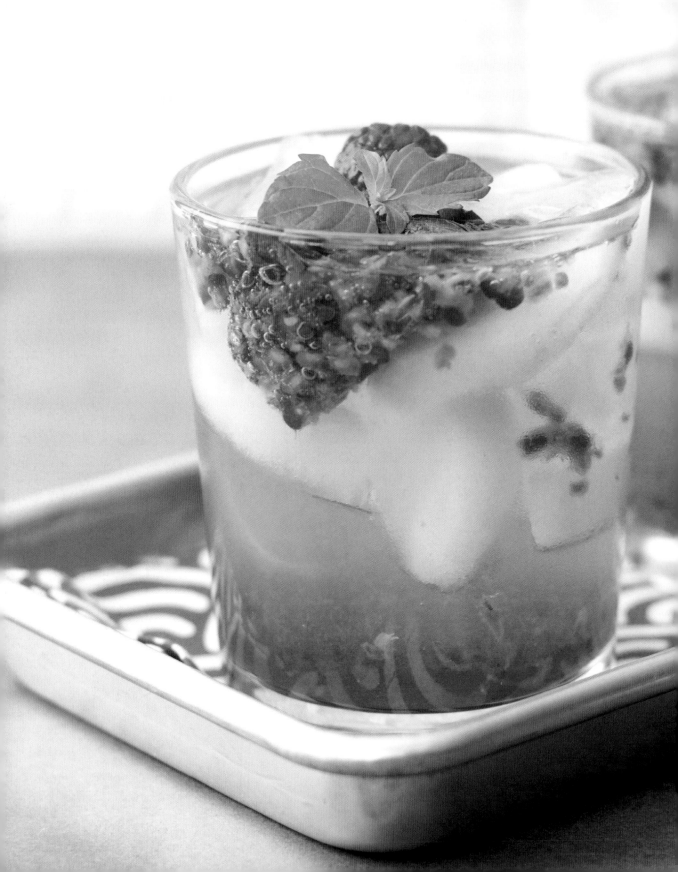

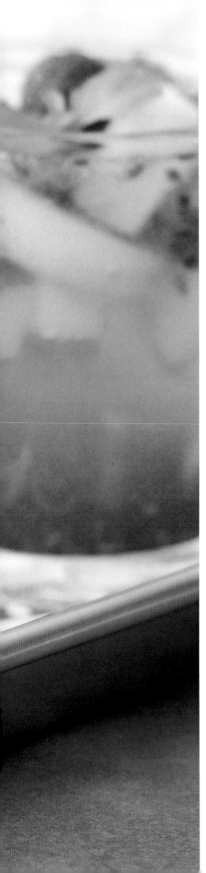

WINE
drinks

NET CARBS
5.7g

Lady in Red

I like to think of this wine cocktail as sort of a lazy sangria. It is super simple to throw together and has all the refreshing characteristics of a scratch-made sangria, but without the extra carbs and sugar. For an even more sangria-like experience, try quadrupling the recipe and serving it in a pitcher with slices of fresh citrus fruits.

Makes 1 drink

6 ounces dry red wine

2 ounces Sweet-and-Sour Mix (page 46)

4 ounces club soda

Lime wheel, for garnish

Lemon half-moon or wedge, for garnish

1 Fill an oversized wine glass with ice. Pour the wine and sweet-and-sour mix over the ice and stir to combine.

2 Top with the club soda and stir gently.

3 Garnish with a lime wheel and a lemon half-moon.

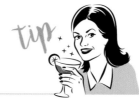

Have some leftover red wine from a couple nights ago? This cocktail is the perfect recipe for red wine that might be approaching the end of its drinkability.

CALORIES: 117 | FAT: 0.1g | PROTEIN: 0.2g | TOTAL CARBS: 5.9g | DIETARY FIBER: 0.2g | NET CARBS: 5.7g | ERYTHRITOL: 12g

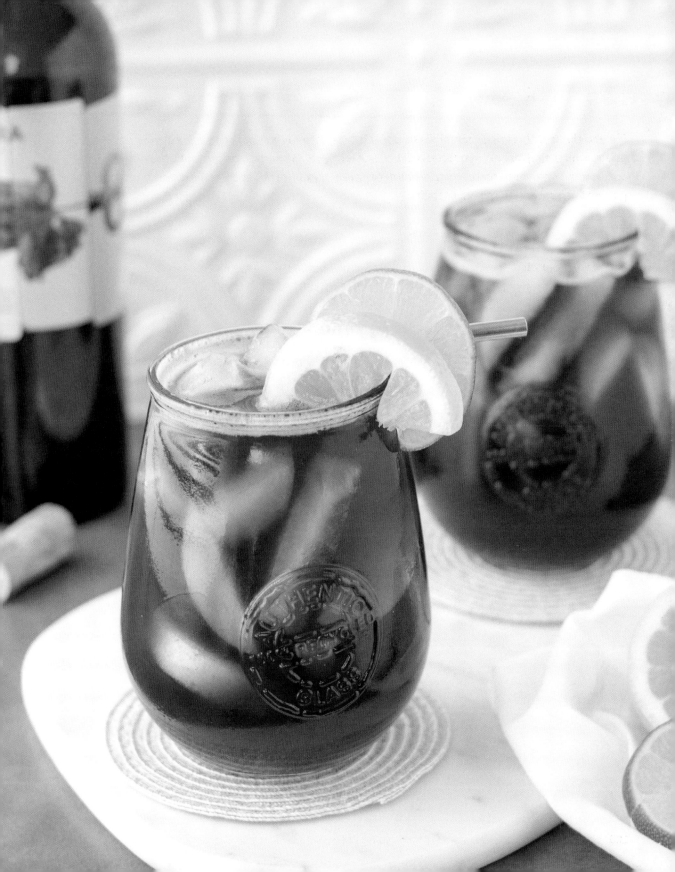

Make It a Mimosa

Mimosas grace the drinks lists of brunch menus everywhere. A mimosa is most commonly made with orange juice, but many of the restaurants in Seattle, where I am from, have entire drinks lists composed solely of mimosa variations. While a typical mimosa has an almost one-to-one ratio of champagne to juice, I prefer to taste the refreshing zing of the bubbles, with just a hint of fruit flavor. Even better, enjoying a mimosa this way keeps the carbs down even more.

Makes 1 drink

5 ounces champagne or prosecco

Splash of fresh grapefruit juice

Grapefruit wedge, for garnish

Pour the sparkling wine into a champagne flute and top with the grapefruit juice. Garnish with a grapefruit wedge.

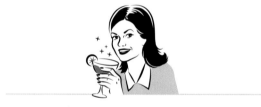

variations

Cranberry Mimosa:
5 ounces champagne or prosecco
Splash of light cranberry juice
A few fresh cranberries, for garnish

Raspberry Mimosa:
5 ounces champagne or prosecco
10 raspberries, blended into a puree, plus more for garnish

Strawberry Mimosa:
5 ounces champagne or prosecco
3 strawberries, hulled and blended into a puree, plus more for garnish

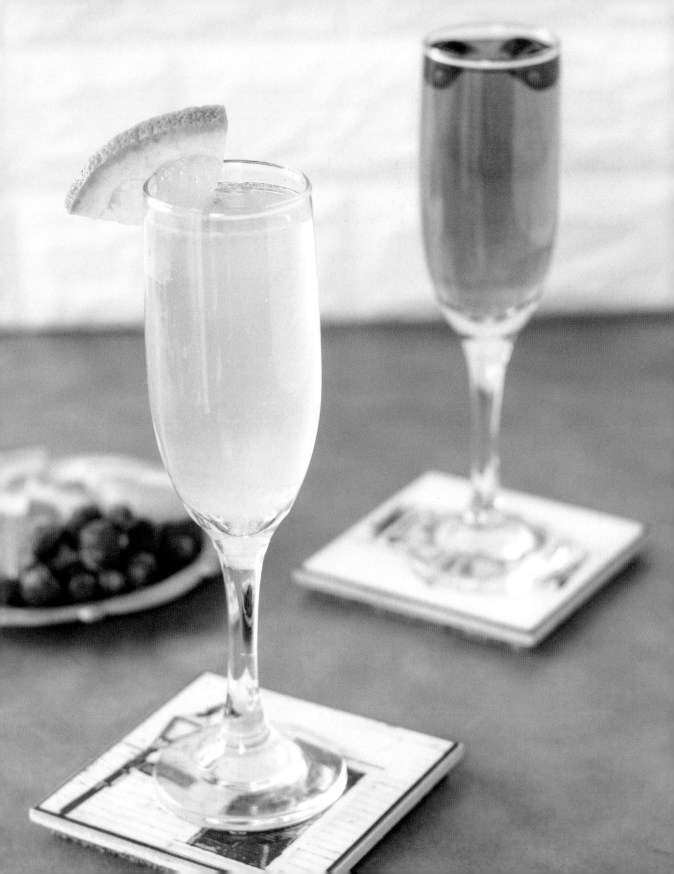

NET CARBS
6g

Mixed Berry
Prosecco Slushie

This is the perfect quick and easy low-carb frozen sparkling wine cocktail. It's delicious after a long day of work or to sip on as you sit next to the pool on a hot summer's day.

Makes 1 drink

½ cup frozen mixed berries

½ ounce vodka

4 ounces prosecco

½ ounce fresh lime juice

¼ cup crushed ice

Lime wheel, for garnish

Combine all the ingredients in a blender and pulse until smooth. Pour into a 16-ounce glass. Garnish with a lime wheel.

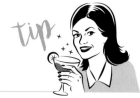

If you prefer a sweeter drink, try adding a little powdered erythritol or Low-Carb Simple Syrup (page 40) to sweeten it.

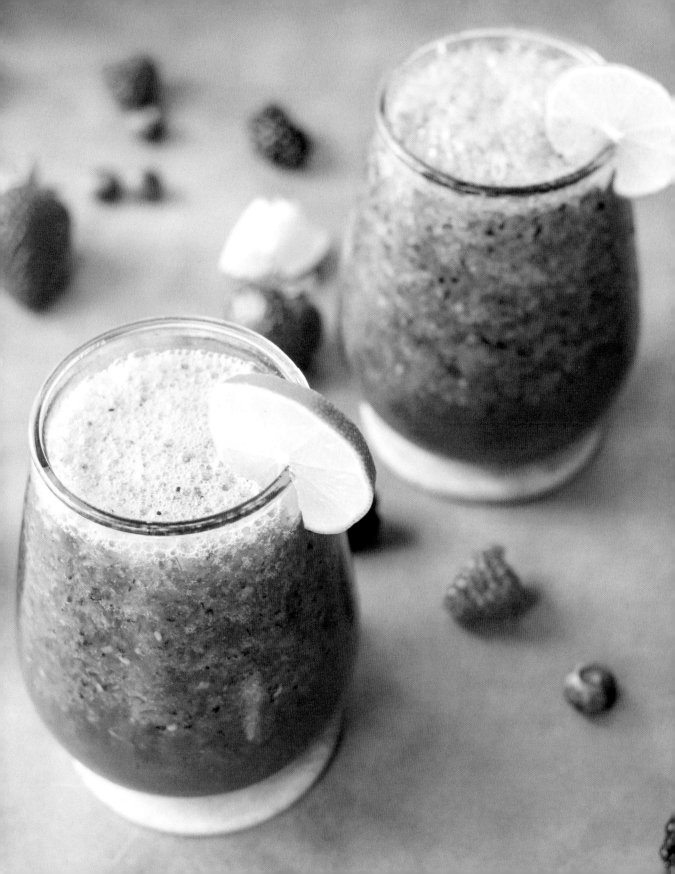

Raspberry-Mint Sparkler

This refreshing sparkling cocktail really shines with the addition of red pepper flakes. Their subtle heat, the tartness of the raspberries, and the sweetness of the simple syrup all come together in perfect harmony.

Makes 1 drink

10 raspberries, plus 1 raspberry for garnish

6 fresh mint leaves, plus 1 small sprig for garnish

Pinch of red pepper flakes

1½ ounces vodka

¼ ounce Low-Carb Simple Syrup (page 40)

4 ounces prosecco

1 Put the raspberries, mint leaves, red pepper flakes, vodka, and simple syrup in a cocktail shaker. Muddle until the raspberries are crushed and have released their juices.

2 Fill a large rocks glass with ice. Pour the raspberry mixture from the cocktail shaker over the ice.

3 Top with the prosecco. Garnish with a small sprig of mint and a raspberry.

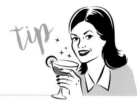

This drink is also delicious with strawberries or blueberries. If using strawberries, slice the tops off of 3 strawberries and thinly slice the berries. If using blueberries, simply substitute 10 blueberries.

CALORIES: 278 | FAT: 0 | PROTEIN: 0 | TOTAL CARBS: 8g | DIETARY FIBER: 1g | NET CARBS: 7g | ERYTHRITOL: 6g

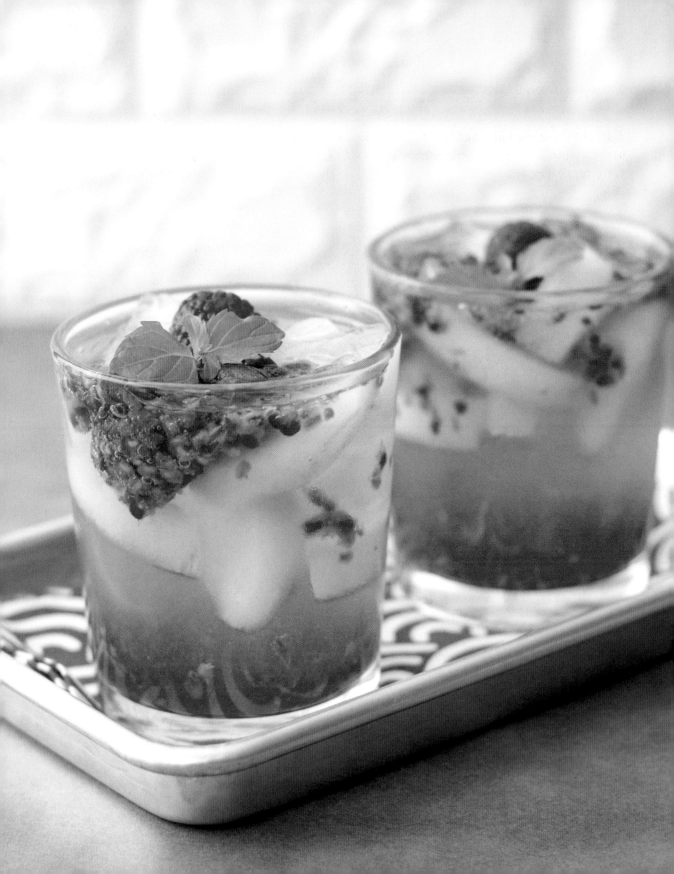

Strawberry Frosé

The Frosé—frozen rosé—is the cocktail equivalent of celebrity couple names: Bennifer, Brangelina, and so on. It's the it drink of summertime girls' nights everywhere.

Makes 1 drink

6 ounces rosé wine

½ cup frozen whole strawberries

½ ounce Low-Carb Simple Syrup (page 40)

½ ounce fresh lemon juice

1 Pour the rosé into a shallow bowl and place it in the freezer for 5 to 6 hours. It won't get completely solid due to the alcohol content, but it will get nice and slushy.

2 Combine the semifrozen rosé, strawberries, simple syrup, and lemon juice in a blender and pulse until smooth and icy. Pour into a Collins glass and serve.

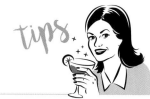

This drink is also delicious made with prosecco.

If you don't want to wait 5 or 6 hours for the wine to chill, or you simply forgot to chill it beforehand, you can add more frozen strawberries to help keep the drink ice-cold and perfectly slushy.

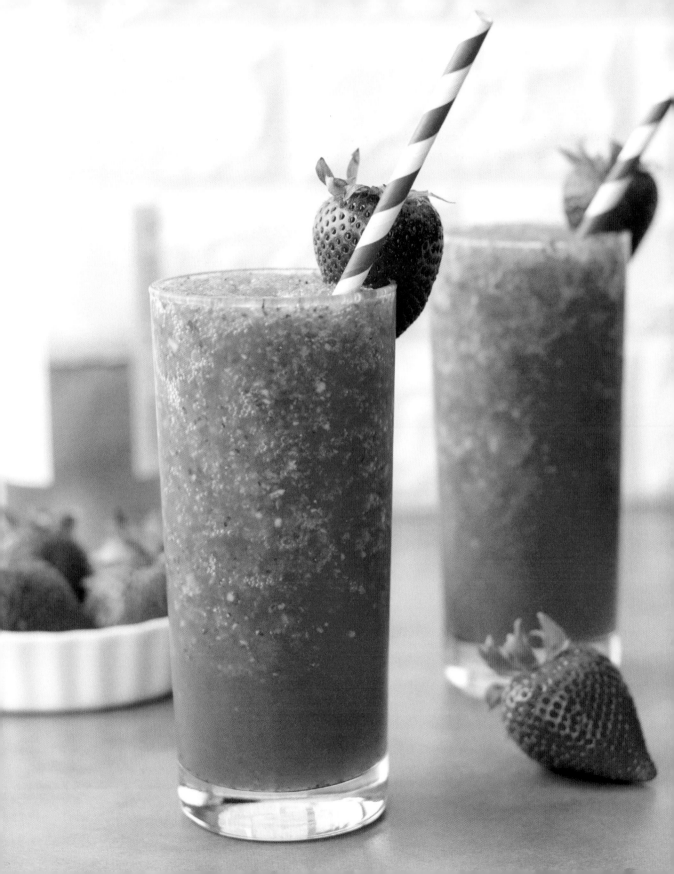

White Wine Spritzer

Back when I was still working in restaurants, every Sunday we would get a group of older ladies wearing big red hats with purple embellishments, and they would all drink white wine spritzers. They were members of the Red Hat Society, a group of women who come together for fun, empowerment, and friendship. I remember asking myself why anyone would want to ruin a perfectly good glass of wine by adding club soda to it . . . until I tried it. The club soda adds an extra refreshing element to an ice-cold glass of white wine on a hot day.

Makes 1 drink

6 ounces ice-cold dry white wine

3 ounces well-chilled club soda

3 raspberries, for garnish (optional)

1 Place the bottle of wine in the freezer for a couple of hours, until it's ice-cold but not slushy. At the same time, have the club soda chilling in the refrigerator.

2 Pour the cold white wine into an oversized wine glass and top with the club soda.

3 Garnish with a few fresh raspberries, if desired.

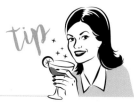

tip

Chilling the wine in the freezer means that you'll need to plan ahead, but it is definitely worth it. I recommend that you make this drink with very, very cold white wine and chilled club soda and serve it without ice, as ice tends to water down the drink. However, if you forget to pop the wine in the freezer beforehand, no worries—simply serve the drink over ice. It will still be refreshing.

CALORIES: 139 | FAT: 0 | PROTEIN: 0 | TOTAL CARBS: 4g | DIETARY FIBER: 0g | NET CARBS: 4g

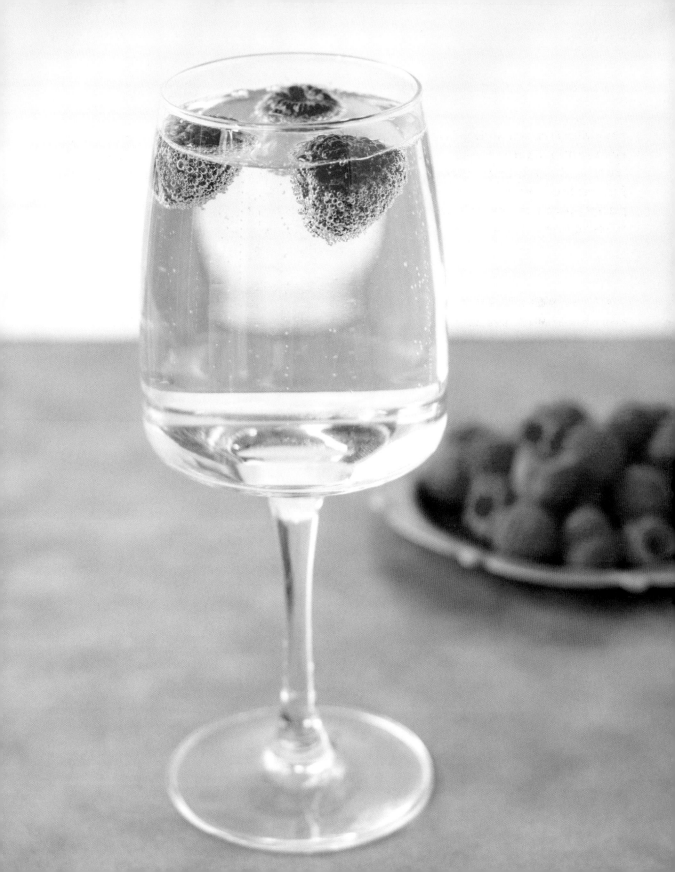

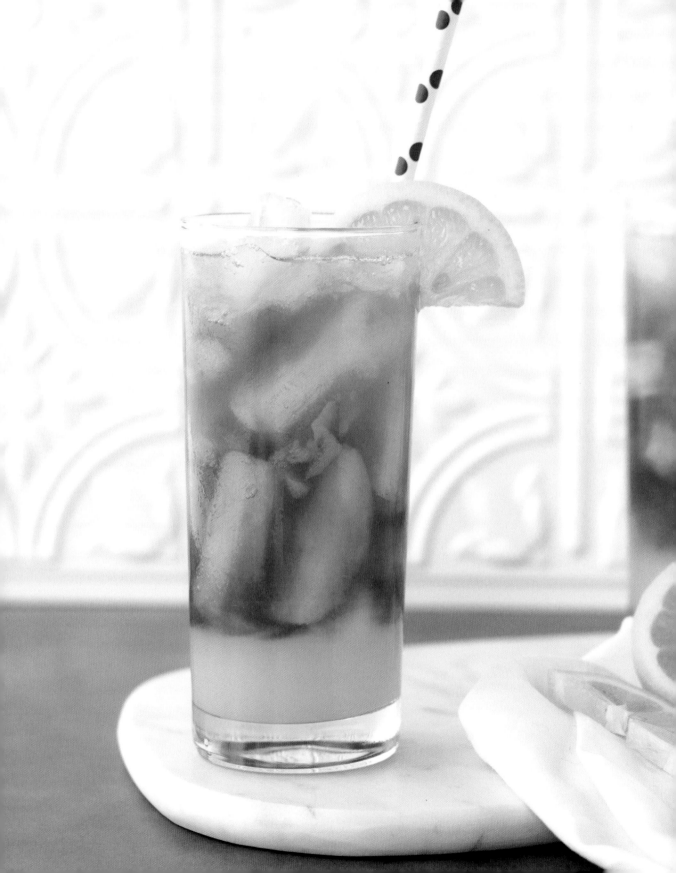

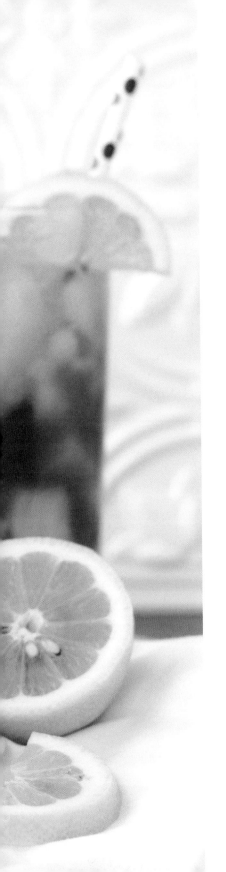

MIXIN' IT *Up*

Espresso Martini

This is one of my favorite after-dinner drinks. Why put alcohol in your coffee when you can put coffee in your alcohol? Of course, there is nothing wrong with loading up a hot cup of delicious dark-roast coffee with homemade Irish cream, either.

Makes 1 drink

½ ounce vodka

1 ounce Homemade Coffee Liqueur (page 166)

1 ounce Homemade Irish Cream Liqueur (page 164)

1 shot espresso

3 espresso beans, for garnish (optional)

1   Fill a cocktail shaker with ice. Add the vodka, coffee liqueur, Irish cream liqueur, and espresso. Cap and shake vigorously.

2   Strain the contents of the cocktail shaker into a chilled martini glass.

3   Garnish with espresso beans, if desired.

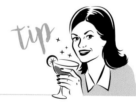

tip

If you are a fan of mochas, try adding a teaspoon of unsweetened cocoa powder and a teaspoon of powdered erythritol for a sweet chocolaty version.

CALORIES: 175 | FAT: 7g | PROTEIN: 0.4g | TOTAL CARBS: 0.5g | DIETARY FIBER: 0 | NET CARBS: 0.5g | ERYTHRITOL: 10g

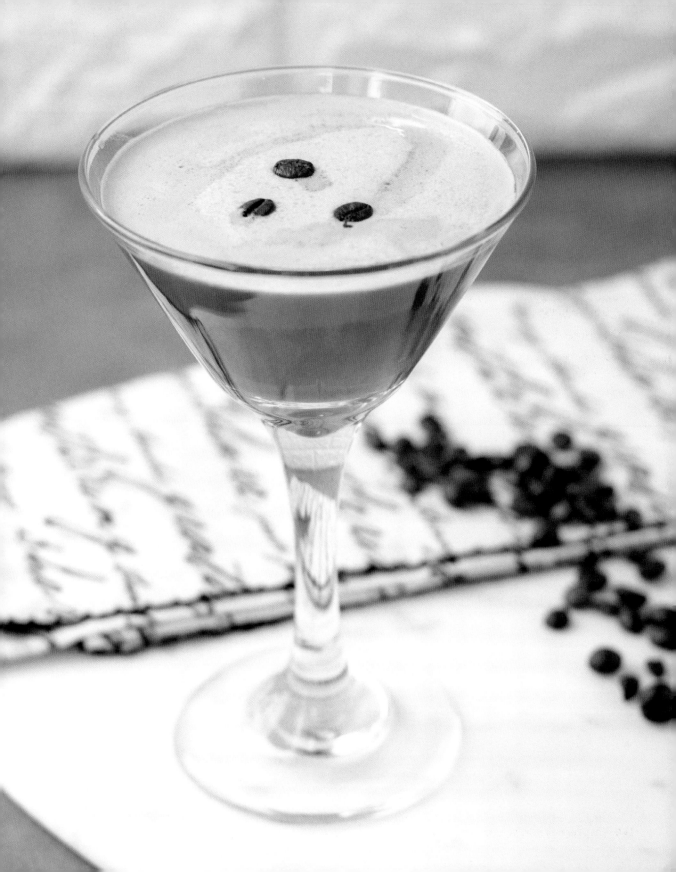

French 75

Like most classic cocktails, the history of this one is a little muddled. However, the one thing that seems to be unanimously agreed upon is that the first printed recipe for the French 75 dates back to a book published in 1930, The Savoy Cocktail Book. *The floral notes of the gin pair perfectly with the bright flavors of fresh citrus. Throw some bubbles into the mix and you have a match made in cocktail heaven.*

Makes 1 drink

1 ounce dry gin

½ ounce fresh lemon juice

1 teaspoon powdered erythritol

4 ounces champagne

Lemon twist, for garnish

1   Combine the gin, lemon juice, and erythritol in a champagne flute and stir.

2   Top with the champagne and garnish with a lemon twist.

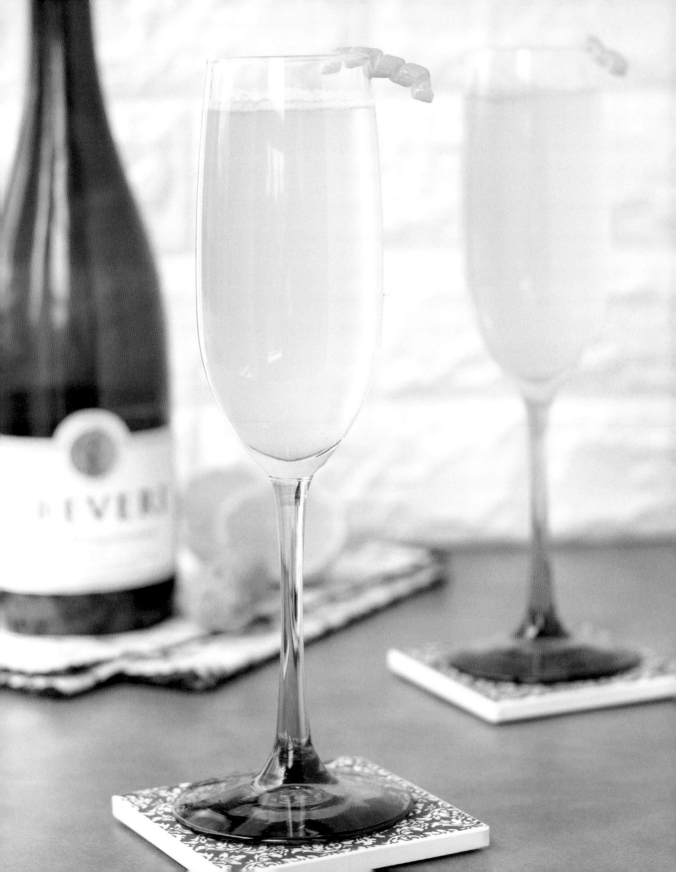

Long Beach Iced Tea

The Long Beach Iced Tea is a lightened-up version of its older, heavier brother, the Long Island Iced Tea. For our trip to Long Beach, we are ditching the cola for a light and fruity cranberry juice floater.

Makes 1 drink

½ ounce vodka

½ ounce white rum

½ ounce dry gin

½ ounce silver tequila

2 ounces Sweet-and-Sour Mix (page 46)

1 ounce light cranberry juice

Lemon wheel or half-moon, for garnish

1   Fill a Collins glass with ice. Pour the vodka, rum, gin, tequila, and sweet-and-sour mix over the ice. Stir to combine.

2   Float the cranberry juice on top.

3   Garnish with a lemon wheel or half-moon.

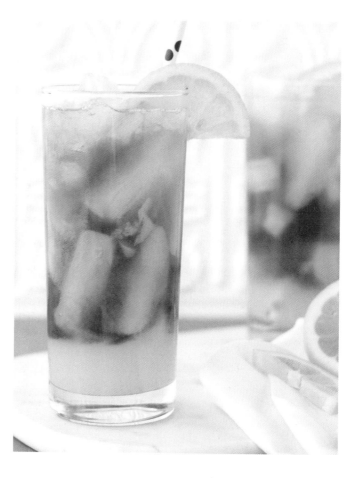

MIXIN'
IT UP

NET CARBS
6g

Whiskey Sunset

Move over, Tequila Sunrise; there's a new drink in town, and it's the Whiskey Sunset. The beautifully layered colors of this drink remind me of the sun setting over Maui—my favorite place! If red wine isn't your thing, try making this cocktail with white wine instead. It's equally refreshing.

Makes 1 drink

2 ounces whiskey

1½ ounces fresh lemon juice

⅓ ounce Low-Carb Simple Syrup (page 40)

4 ounces dry red wine

Lemon wheel, for garnish

Fresh cherry, for garnish

1 Pour the whiskey, lemon juice, and simple syrup into an oversized wine glass. Stir to combine.

2 Fill the glass with ice and top with the red wine.

3 Garnish with a lemon wheel and a cherry.

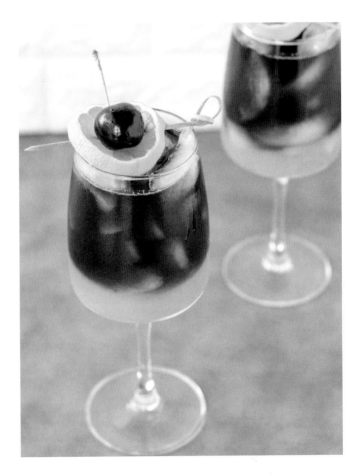

CALORIES: 239 | FAT: 0 | PROTEIN: 0 | TOTAL CARBS: 6g | DIETARY FIBER: 0 | NET CARBS: 6g | ERYTHRITOL: 9g

NET CARBS
0.8g

Landslide

The Landslide is my low-carb take on the ever-popular Mudslide. It is delicious on ice, blended, or even in coffee. When you combine Irish cream, coffee liqueur, and vodka, you can't really go wrong.

Makes 1 drink

1½ ounces Homemade Irish Cream Liqueur (page 164)

1 ounce Homemade Coffee Liqueur (page 166)

1 ounce vodka

Fill a cocktail shaker with ice. Add the Irish cream, coffee liqueur, and vodka. Cap and shake vigorously. Pour the contents of the shaker into a 12-ounce glass.

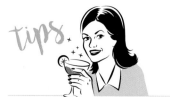

tips

For a fun frozen version, try mixing this with a scoop of low-carb vanilla ice cream in a blender. Or, for a creamier shaken version, try adding some Fresh Whipped Cream (page 47) to the cocktail shaker.

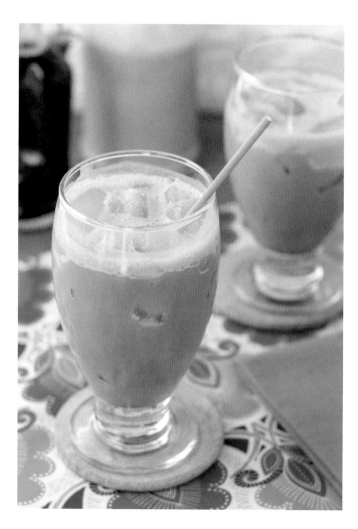

Black Russian

The Black Russian is so named because it includes the quintessential Russian spirit, vodka. The "black" part comes into play with the dark, bold colors of the coffee liqueur. For a lighter, creamy version, try the abiding White Russian (page 148).

Makes 1 drink

1½ ounces vodka

1 ounce Homemade Coffee Liqueur (page 166)

Fresh cherry, for garnish (optional)

Fill a rocks glass with ice. Pour the vodka and coffee liqueur over the ice. Garnish with a cherry, if desired.

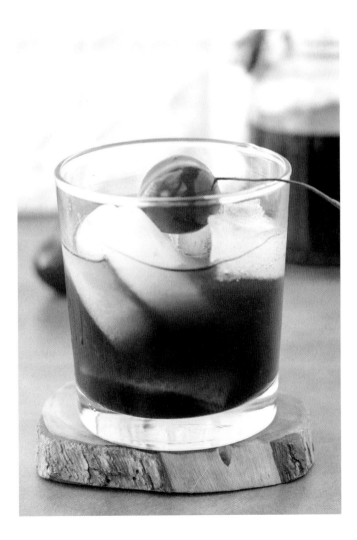

White Russian

Like the Dude, the White Russian abides. I love how many cocktails can instantly bring up memories of favorite movies and television shows. This drink was repopularized by the Dude in the movie The Big Lebowski. *Don't let this simple three-ingredient drink fool you—it certainly doesn't skimp on flavor. "Careful, man, there's a beverage here!" —The Dude*

Makes 1 drink

2 ounces Homemade Coffee Liqueur (page 166)

1½ ounces vodka

1½ ounces heavy cream

Fill a large rocks glass with ice. Pour the coffee liqueur and vodka over the ice. Top with the heavy cream.

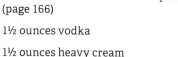

This drink is delicious with a splash of Homemade Irish Cream Liqueur (page 164).

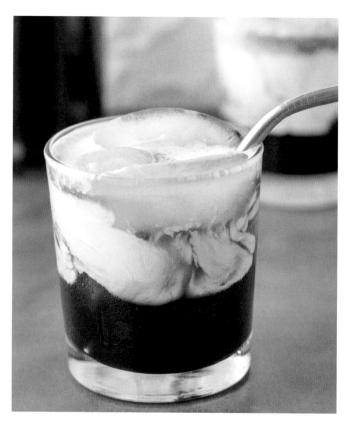

Winearita

Red wine and tequila—have I gone mad? If by "mad" you mean "madly in love with this drink," then yes, I have in fact gone mad. This drink fusion is what might result if a glass of sangria met a margarita and they fell in love and lived happily ever after. The boldness of red wine mixed with the smooth bite of tequila and the tang of sweet-and-sour mix really makes this drink come alive.

Makes 1 drink

1½ ounces silver tequila

2 ounces dry red wine

1 ounce Sweet-and-Sour Mix (page 46)

2 drops of pure orange extract

Lime twist, for garnish

1 Fill a cocktail shaker with ice. Add the tequila, wine, sweet-and-sour mix, and orange extract. Cap and shake vigorously.

2 Strain the contents of the cocktail shaker into a chilled margarita glass.

3 Garnish with a lime twist.

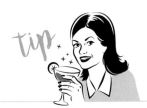

tip

If you are not a fan of tequila, try making this drink with spiced rum.

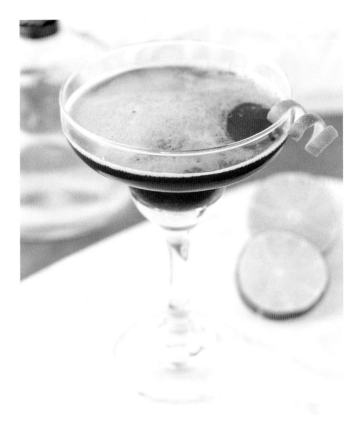

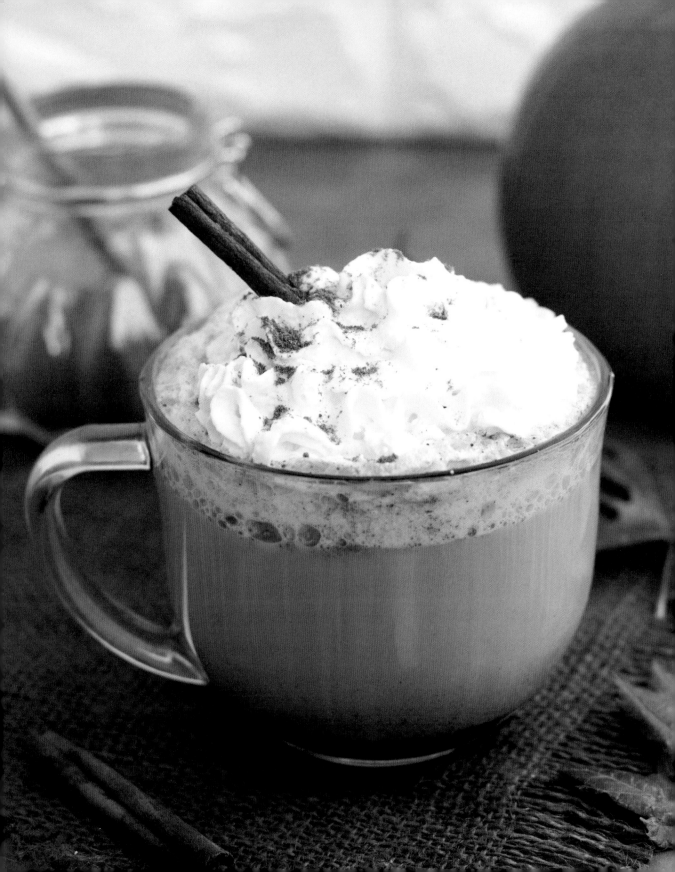

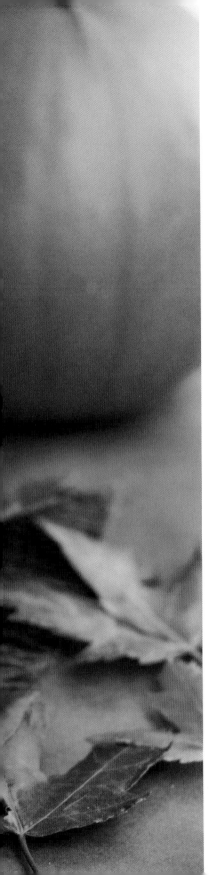

CHAPTER 9

HOT DRINKS AND *Cordials*

Boosted and Spiked Pumpkin Spice Latte

Fall's favorite latte gets kicked up a notch in this boosted and spiked version. You've no doubt heard of butter coffee or boosted coffee. Why not take it to the next level with a little bit of pumpkin pie spice and some spiced rum?

Makes 1 drink

2 ounces spiced rum

12 ounces freshly brewed hot coffee

1 tablespoon plus 1 teaspoon sugar-free salted caramel syrup, or more to taste

1 tablespoon heavy cream, or more to make it creamier

1 tablespoon salted butter

2 tablespoons grass-fed collagen peptides

1 teaspoon pumpkin pie spice, plus more for garnish

Fresh Whipped Cream (page 47) (optional)

Cinnamon stick, for garnish (optional)

1   Pour the rum into a large coffee mug.

2   Combine the coffee, caramel syrup, cream, butter, collagen peptides, and pumpkin pie spice in a blender or milk frother and blend until creamy.

3   Pour the coffee mixture into the mug with the rum and top with whipped cream, if using, and a sprinkle of pumpkin pie spice. Garnish with a cinnamon stick, if desired.

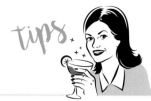

tips

When shopping for flavored sugar-free syrups, look for brands that are sweetened with erythritol.

If you do not have collagen peptides on hand, you can simply omit it. It is used to boost the nutritional value of this drink by adding all the healthy benefits of collagen.

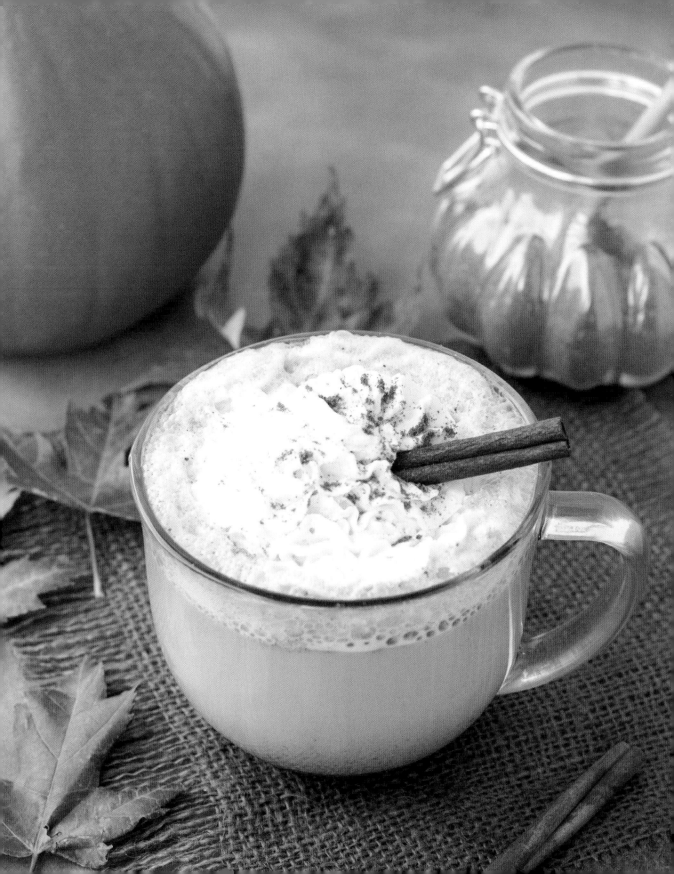

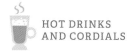

Boozy Hot Cocoa

It's time to take your favorite childhood winter treat to a new level. The flavors of Irish cream and coffee liqueur are a match made in heaven when combined with delicious hot cocoa. Top it with some fresh whipped cream and grated dark chocolate and you have a low-carb dream come true. I dare you to drink only one!

Makes 1 drink

1 ounce Homemade Coffee Liqueur (page 166)

1 ounce Homemade Irish Cream Liqueur (page 164)

6 ounces sugar-free, low-carb hot cocoa (see tips)

2 tablespoons Fresh Whipped Cream (page 47)

Grated or shaved sugar-free dark chocolate, for garnish (optional)

Put the liqueurs and hot cocoa in a coffee mug. Stir to combine. Top with whipped cream and grated or shaved chocolate, if using.

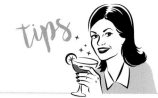

tips

This drink is also amazing with hot coffee!

You can make your own hot cocoa from scratch using unsweetened cocoa powder, a keto-friendly sweetener, such as erythritol, and a low-carb milk substitute, such as unsweetened almond or coconut milk. For an even creamier version, you can make it with heavy cream.

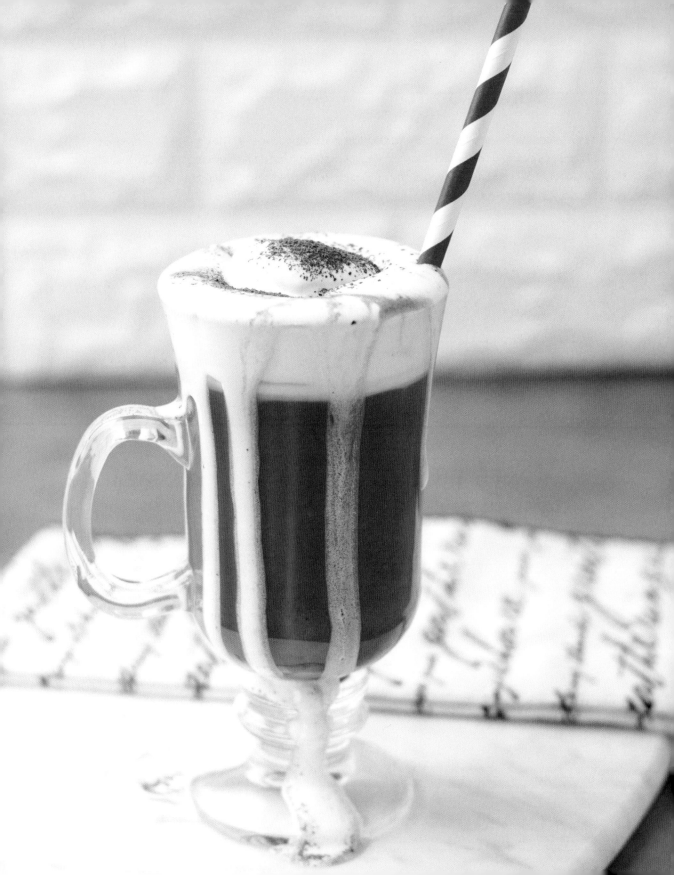

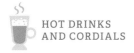

Coffee-Spiked Coffee

Adding coffee liqueur to coffee might sound a little redundant, but it is the perfect way to spike your favorite morning beverage. It adds a hint of sweetness and a nice toasted flavor. If you are not a coffee drinker, try making this drink with a sugar-free, low-carb hot cocoa mix.

Makes 1 drink

2 ounces Homemade Coffee Liqueur
(page 166)

5 ounces freshly brewed hot coffee

Fresh Whipped Cream (page 47)
(optional)

In a coffee mug, combine the liqueur and coffee. Top with whipped cream, if desired.

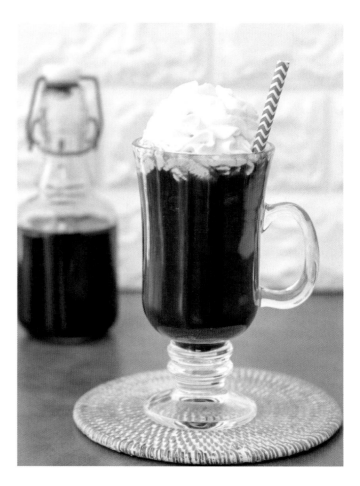

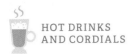
Hot Toddy

Whether you are looking to warm up on a cold winter's day or to get into a festive holiday spirit, this is the drink for you. Many people also swear by drinking a Hot Toddy when they are feeling under the weather, reporting that it helps with nasal congestion and the sniffles. I like to think of it as a sort of boozy Theraflu.

Makes 1 drink

2 ounces whiskey

8 ounces hot water

1 tablespoon fresh lemon juice

2 teaspoons powdered erythritol

Pinch of ground cloves

Pinch of ground nutmeg

Cinnamon stick

Lemon wheel

Combine all the ingredients in a large coffee mug. Let the cinnamon and lemon steep in the hot liquid for a few minutes before enjoying.

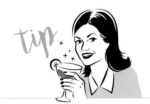

For a delicious tea variation, try adding a bag of orange spice or Earl Grey tea.

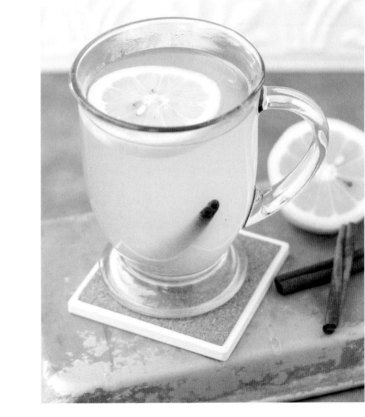

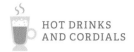
Flameless Mexican Coffee

There are a lot of different variations of Mexican coffee, but the one I see the most involves torching the sugared rim to caramelize it and then melting vanilla ice cream into the drink. I decided to go for a flameless version, as we don't need any kitchen accidents during cocktail hour. In place of ice cream, I used fresh whipped cream to create that beautifully frothy foam on top.

Makes 1 drink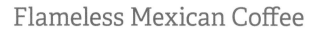

8 ounces freshly brewed hot coffee, divided

1 tablespoon granular erythritol

¼ teaspoon ground cinnamon

1 ounce silver tequila

1 ounce Homemade Coffee Liqueur (page 166)

2 tablespoons Fresh Whipped Cream (page 47)

TO RIM THE MUG:

1   Pour about 1 tablespoon of the brewed coffee onto a small plate.

2   Pour the erythritol onto a separate small plate. Sprinkle the cinnamon on top of the erythritol.

3   Swirl the rim of a large coffee mug in the coffee, then swirl it in the cinnamon and erythritol to coat the rim.

TO MAKE THE DRINK:

1   Pour the tequila, liqueur, and remaining hot coffee into the rimmed coffee mug.

2   Stir the whipped cream into the drink.

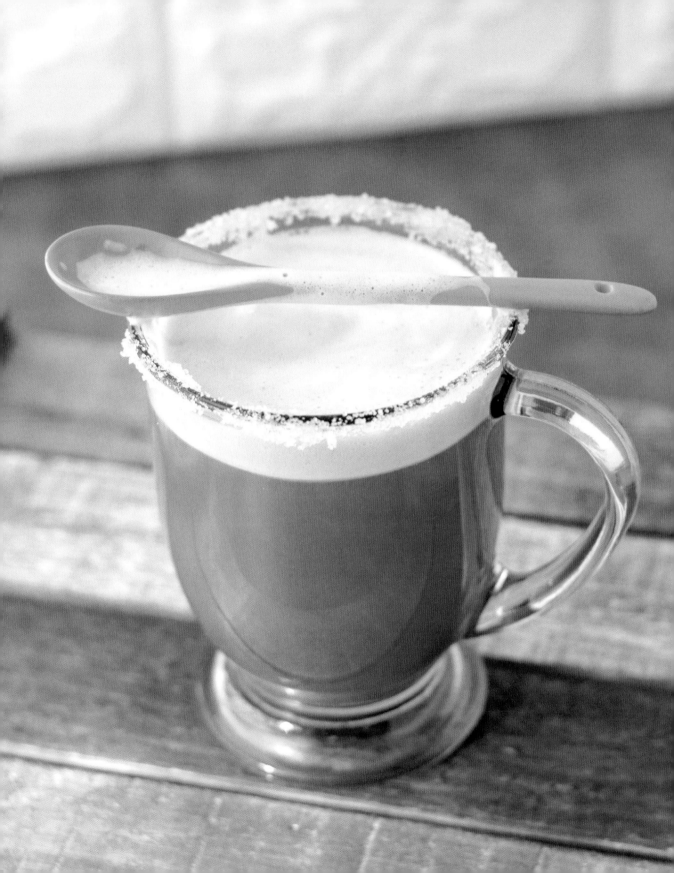

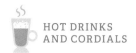

Hot Buttered Rum

This drink is a nod to my childhood. That may sound really strange given that it is an alcoholic beverage, but hear me out. Along with the hustle and bustle of family visiting, feasting, and opening presents, we had a couple other Christmas traditions in our home. After the festivities wound down for the evening, all the adults would gather around the table, play games, and drink hot buttered rum. I was so excited when I was finally old enough to take part. To this day, we still uphold this tradition.

Makes 1 drink

2 ounces spiced rum

4 ounces hot water

2 to 3 tablespoons Hot Buttered Rum Mix (opposite)

Fresh Whipped Cream (page 47) (optional)

1 Combine the spiced rum, hot water, and hot buttered rum mix in a coffee mug and stir until the rum mix is dissolved.

2 Top with whipped cream, if desired.

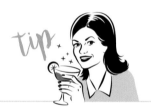

tip

You can also make this drink with dark or light rum.

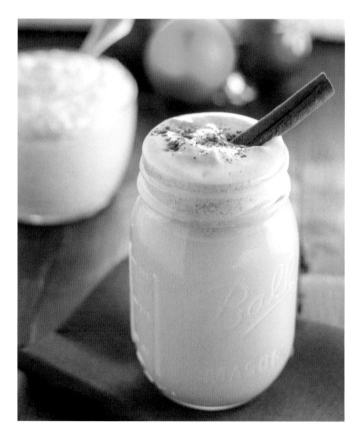

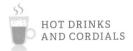
Hot Buttered Rum Mix

If you have ever had hot buttered rum, then you know that the mix used to make it contains a lot of sugar. In an attempt to keep the holidays merry and bright without diving face-first into a glass of sugar, I decided it was high time to make my own low-carb hot buttered rum mix.

Makes 4½ cups (3 tablespoons per serving)

1 cup salted butter

1 cup granular erythritol

3 tablespoons sugar-free maple syrup

1 teaspoon pure vanilla extract

1 cup heavy cream

1½ cups powdered erythritol

¼ teaspoon ground cinnamon

¼ teaspoon ground nutmeg

⅛ teaspoon ground cloves

1　In a large mixing bowl, using a hand mixer on medium speed, cream the butter, granular erythritol, maple syrup, and vanilla extract until the mixture is light and fluffy, about 3 minutes.

2　Add the cream, powdered erythritol, cinnamon, nutmeg, and cloves. Mix on low speed until the ingredients are well combined and the mixture is smooth.

3　Store the mix in an airtight container in the fridge for up to 1 week. After that, transfer it to the freezer, where it will keep indefinitely.

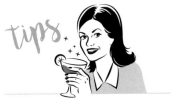

When shopping for flavored sugar-free syrups, look for brands that are sweetened with erythritol.

Hot buttered rum mix makes a great Christmas gift. Whip up a batch, portion it out into small mason jars, and give it with a pint of spiced rum. Start your own holiday hot buttered rum tradition!

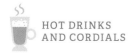

NET CARBS
0.5g

Irish Coffee

Picture this: snow is falling, the fire is crackling, and you are curled up in your favorite chair, wrapped in your fuzziest blanket. Doesn't that sound dreamy? Now imagine that same scenario, but with a delicious hot cocktail in your hand. Perfection! Drinking an Irish Coffee is one of my favorite ways to stay warm in winter.

Makes 1 drink

1 ounce Homemade Irish Cream Liqueur (page 164)

1 ounce Irish whiskey

1 teaspoon brown sugar erythritol (optional)

6 ounces freshly brewed hot coffee

2 tablespoons Fresh Whipped Cream (page 47) (optional)

Shaved or grated sugar-free dark chocolate, for garnish (optional)

1 Put the liqueur, whiskey, and erythritol, if using, in a coffee mug. Stir to combine.

2 Add the coffee and stir.

3 Top with whipped cream and chocolate shavings, if desired.

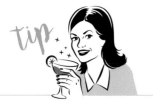

tip

This drink is also great with sugar-free, low-carb hot cocoa.

CALORIES: 149 | FAT: 7g | PROTEIN: 0.4g | TOTAL CARBS: 0.5g | DIETARY FIBER: 0 | NET CARBS: 0.5g | ERYTHRITOL: 2g

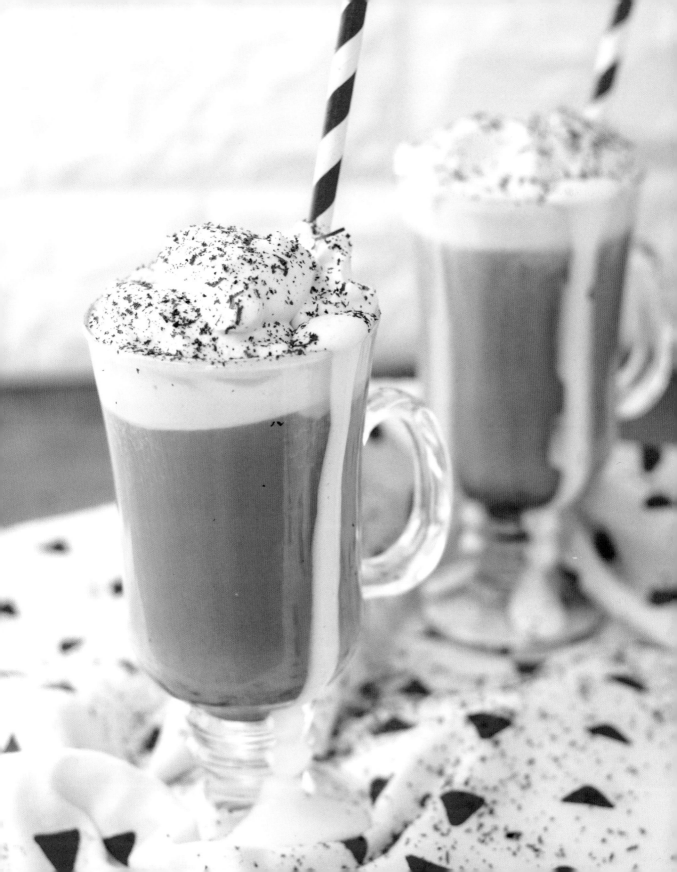

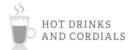

Homemade
Irish Cream Liqueur

Move over, Baileys; there's a low-carb Irish cream in town, and it is delicious! This liqueur is equally enjoyable served on the rocks or in coffee.

Makes 28 ounces (2 ounces per serving)

2 cups heavy cream

1 cup Irish whiskey

⅔ cup powdered erythritol

2 teaspoons unsweetened cocoa powder

1 teaspoon instant espresso granules

1 teaspoon pure almond extract

1 teaspoon pure vanilla extract

Combine all the ingredients in a blender and pulse until well combined. Store in the refrigerator for up to 1 month.

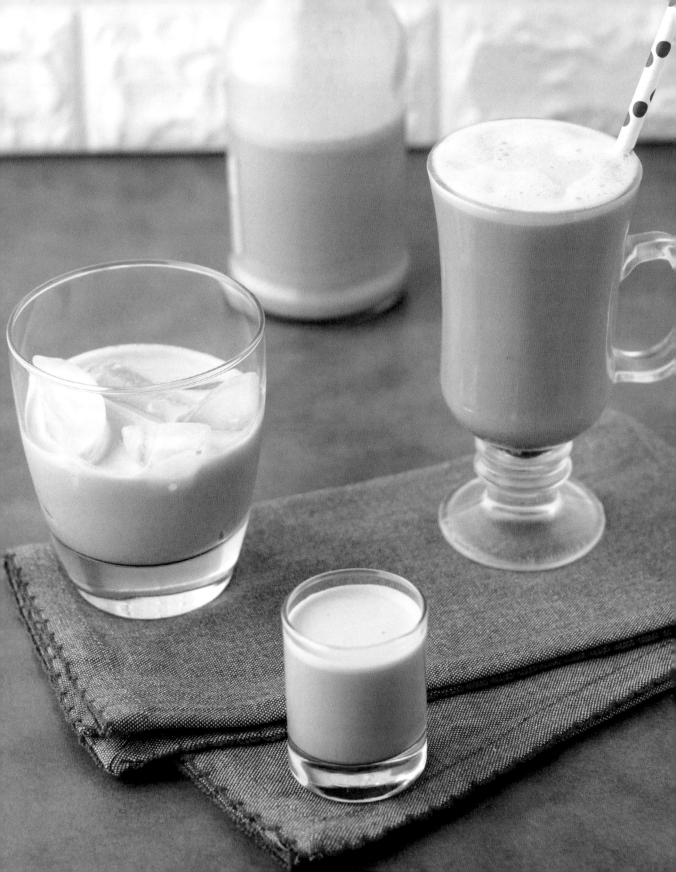

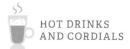

Homemade Coffee Liqueur

This is my homemade low-carb nod to Kahlúa. Back in my high-carb, high-sugar days, Kahlúa was one of my go-to winter liqueurs. Combine this version with Homemade Irish Cream Liqueur (page 164) and you have a match made in heaven, perfect for iced drinks and hot drinks alike.

Makes 24 ounces (2 ounces per serving)

1 cup water

1 cup powdered erythritol

¼ cup plus 2 tablespoons instant espresso granules

1 cup vodka

2 tablespoons pure vanilla extract

1   Bring the water to a boil in a medium saucepan over high heat. Mix in the erythritol and espresso. Reduce the heat to low and whisk until the erythritol and espresso granules dissolve. Remove the pan from the heat and let stand until cool, about 1 hour.

2   Mix the vodka and vanilla extract into the cooled espresso mixture.

3   Transfer the liqueur to a large jar. Seal and store, away from light, for 4 to 6 weeks before drinking.

4   Store in the pantry for up to 6 months. Shake before using.

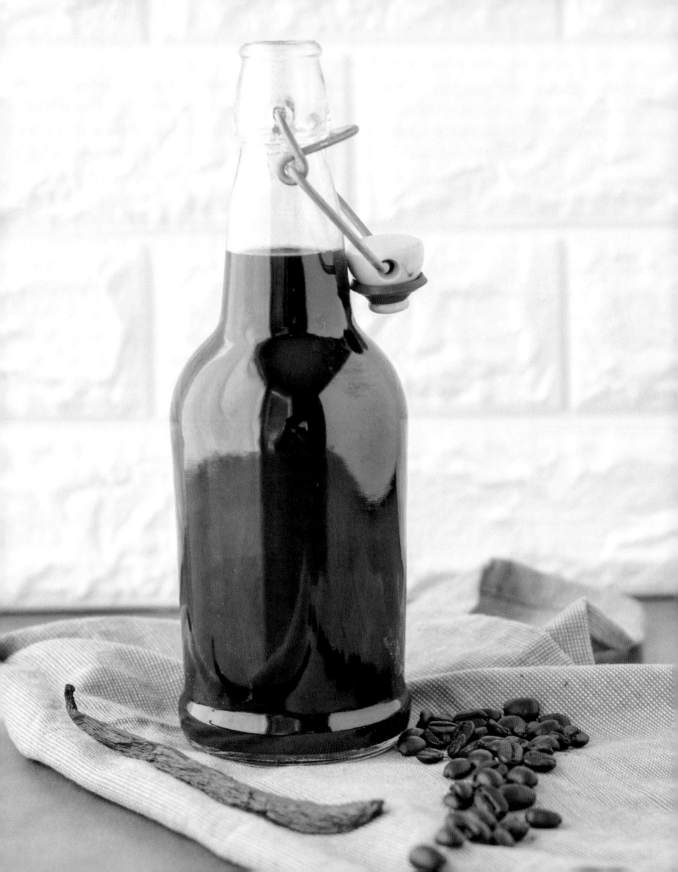

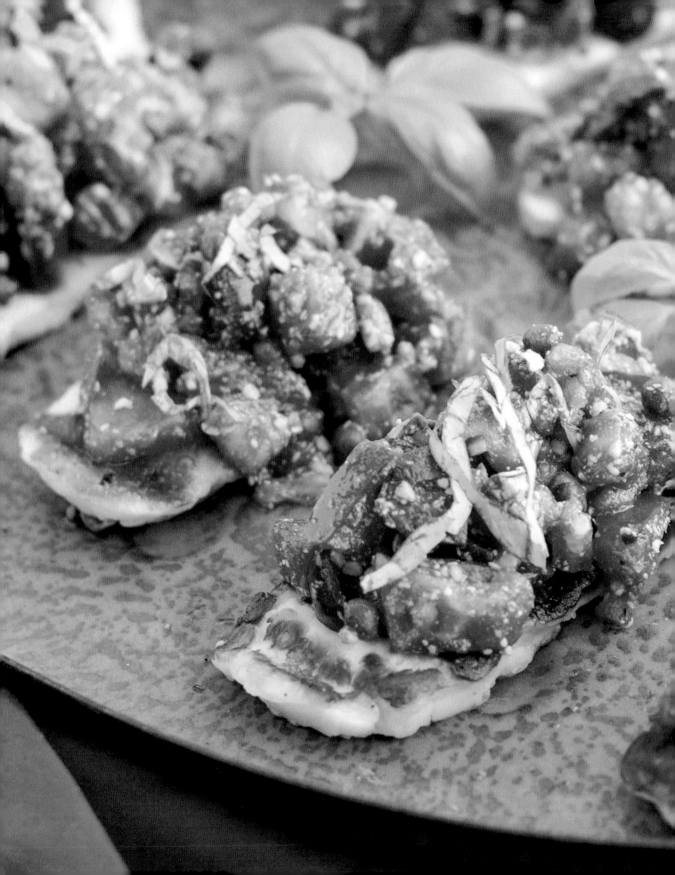

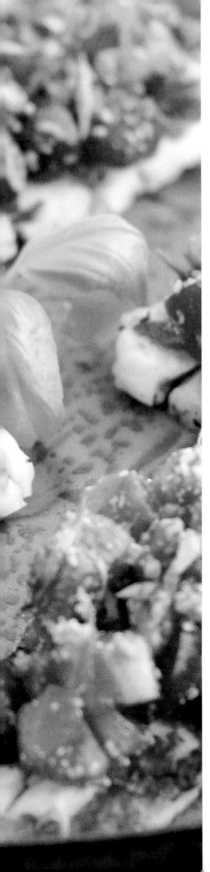
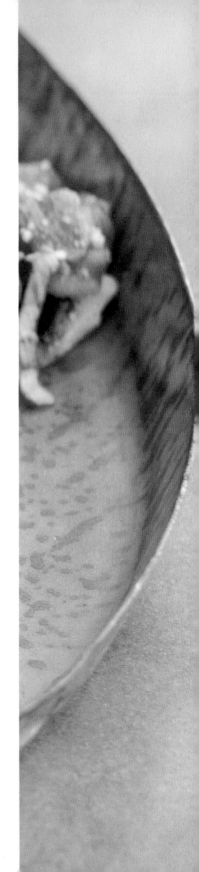

— CHAPTER 10 —

EATS
AND
Treats

Antipasto Salad

This salad is my go-to dish to bring to parties or to serve when I entertain at my house. It has a little something for everyone in it, and with all its beautiful colors, it looks as good as it tastes.

Makes 8 servings | Prep time: 15 minutes

FOR THE DRESSING:

½ cup mayonnaise

1 clove garlic, minced

2 tablespoons balsamic vinegar

FOR THE SALAD:

4 ounces raw cauliflower, cored and cut into small florets

4 ounces sharp cheddar cheese, cubed

2½ ounces sliced pepperoni, quartered

2½ ounces sliced salami, quartered

⅓ cup sliced black olives

1 mini seedless cucumber, quartered lengthwise and then sliced crosswise

10 grape tomatoes, halved

1   Make the dressing: Put the mayonnaise, garlic, and vinegar in a small bowl and whisk to combine.

2   Make the salad: Put all the salad ingredients in a large bowl and toss to combine.

3   Serve the salad with the dressing on the side. Store leftover salad and dressing in separate containers in the refrigerator for up to 1 week.

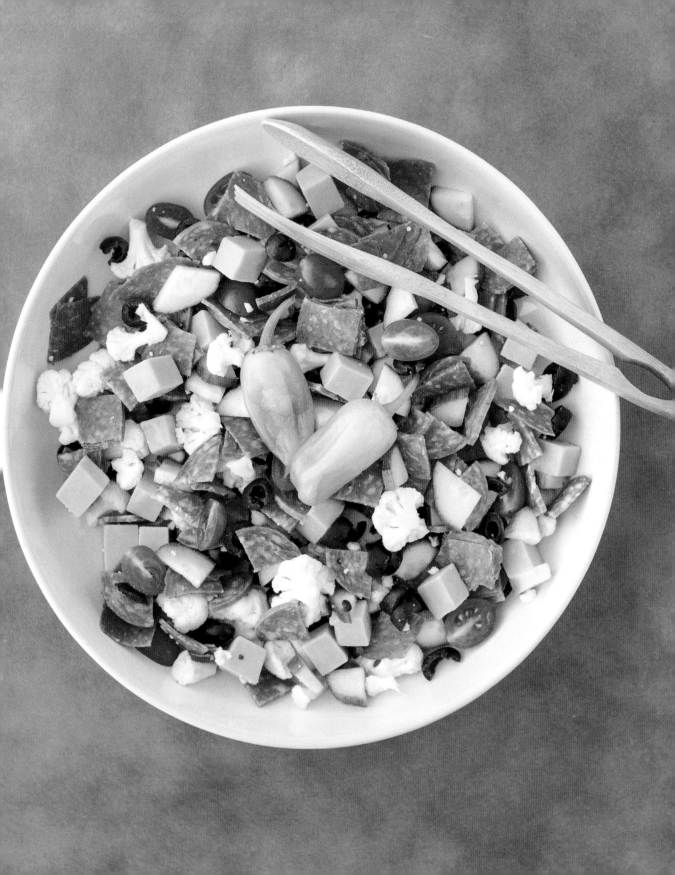

Avocado Hummus

Hummus has always been one of my favorite appetizers, but chickpeas are relatively high in carbs. In this recipe, I use zucchini in place of chickpeas to make a delicious low-carb version. The avocado is a no-brainer, because let's face it, avocado makes just about everything better, am I right?

Makes 10 servings (¼ cup per serving) | Prep time: 15 minutes _____

1 large zucchini, peeled and cubed

1 medium avocado, peeled, pitted, and cubed

Juice of ½ lemon

3 cloves garlic, minced

¼ cup roasted tahini

1 tablespoon avocado oil

1 teaspoon ground cumin

1 teaspoon fine sea salt

Finely diced bell peppers (assorted colors), for garnish (optional)

Raw vegetable dippers of choice, for serving

1 Combine the zucchini, avocado, lemon juice, garlic, tahini, oil, cumin, and salt in a food processor and pulse until smooth and creamy.

2 Refrigerate for at least 1 hour to allow the flavors to come together.

3 Garnish with diced bell peppers, if using, and serve with the vegetable dippers of your choice.

4 Store leftovers in the refrigerator for up to 1 week.

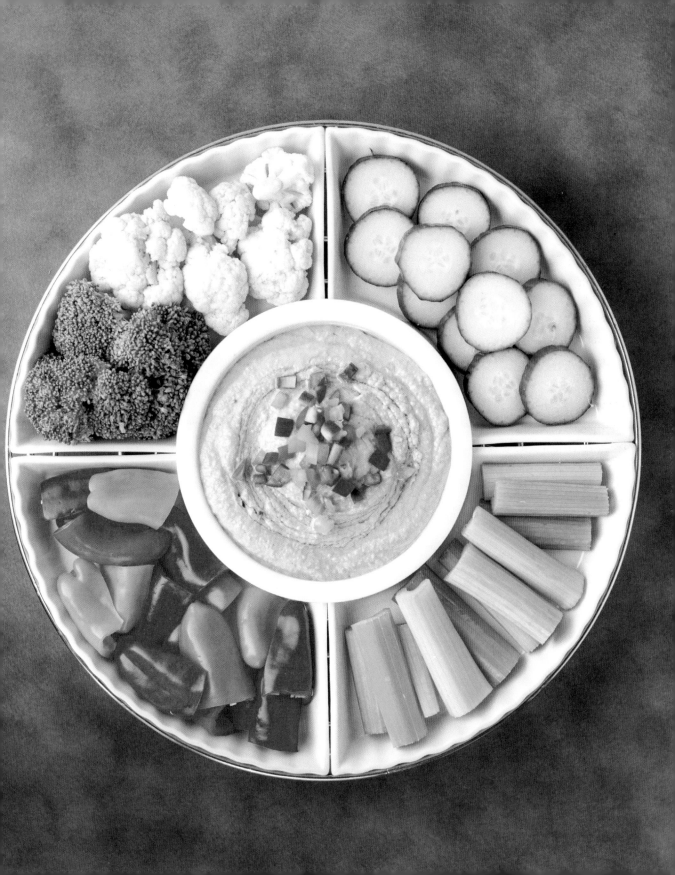

Bacon and Blue Cheese Deviled Eggs

Nature's perfect food just got a delicious upgrade. For this recipe, and for a lot of my deviled egg recipes, I leave the yolks intact. I love getting to experience the rich, creamy texture of a perfectly cooked egg while also tasting the amazing flavors of the mixture piled on top. I think that once you try this recipe, you may just change the way you make your deviled eggs.

Makes 6 deviled eggs (1 per serving) | Prep time: 15 minutes | Cook time: 15 minutes _____

3 large eggs, hard-boiled and peeled (see tip)

¼ cup mayonnaise

1 tablespoon plus 1 teaspoon crumbled blue cheese, plus more for garnish

½ teaspoon chopped fresh chives, plus more for garnish

½ teaspoon chopped fresh dill weed, plus more for garnish

½ teaspoon dried minced onions

¼ teaspoon garlic powder

Pinch of fine sea salt

2 slices bacon, cooked crisp and crumbled

1   Slice the eggs in half, leaving the yolks in the center.

2   In a mixing bowl, mix together the mayonnaise, blue cheese, chives, dill, onions, garlic powder, and salt until well combined.

3   Transfer the mixture to a pastry bag or a resealable plastic bag. If using a resealable plastic bag, snip off one corner of the bag. Pipe the mixture onto the egg halves.

4   Garnish with the bacon and extra blue cheese, chives, and dill.

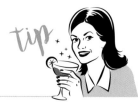

tip

This is how I make perfect hard-boiled eggs: Place the eggs in large saucepan. Add enough water to fully submerge the eggs. Over high heat, bring the water to a rolling boil. Once the water is boiling, remove the pan from the heat, cover, and let sit for 12 minutes. Remove the eggs and submerge them in a cold-water bath before peeling.

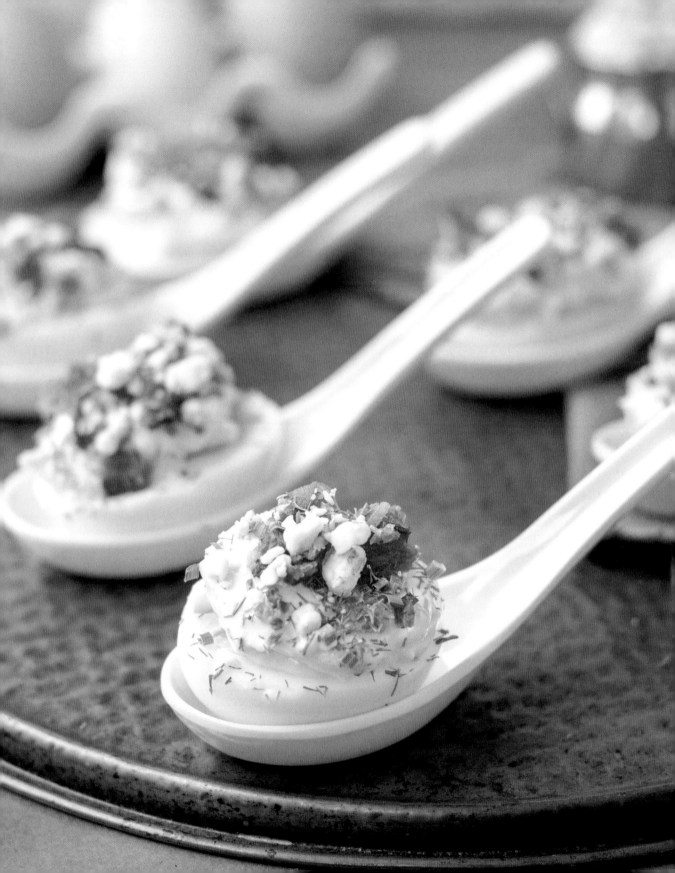

EATS AND
TREATS

Barbecue Cocktail Sausages

Cocktail parties, get-togethers, and potlucks all seem to have one thing in common: you can always count on walking into the kitchen and seeing a delicious dish of cocktail sausages in barbecue sauce. That becomes problematic for those living a low-carb lifestyle, though, because traditional barbecue sauces are very high in sugar and carbs. This recipe solves that problem.

Makes 10 servings | Prep time: 10 minutes | Cook time: 25 minutes _____

1 cup tomato sauce

1 tablespoon salted butter

1½ teaspoons apple cider vinegar

1½ teaspoons liquid smoke

1 teaspoon fresh lemon juice

1 clove garlic, minced

3 tablespoons powdered erythritol

2 teaspoons onion powder

¼ teaspoon fine sea salt

¼ teaspoon ground black pepper

1 pound smoked beef cocktail sausages

1 Combine the tomato sauce, butter, vinegar, liquid smoke, lemon juice, garlic, erythritol, onion powder, salt, and pepper in a saucepan over medium heat. Simmer for 10 minutes.

2 Add the cocktail sausages to the saucepan and simmer for an additional 15 minutes.

3 Taste and add more salt, if desired, before serving.

4 Store leftovers in the refrigerator for up to 1 week.

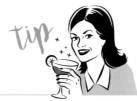

Instead of preparing these sausages on the stovetop, you can combine all the ingredients in a slow cooker and cook on low for 6 hours. This is a great option if you are making this dish to take to a gathering.

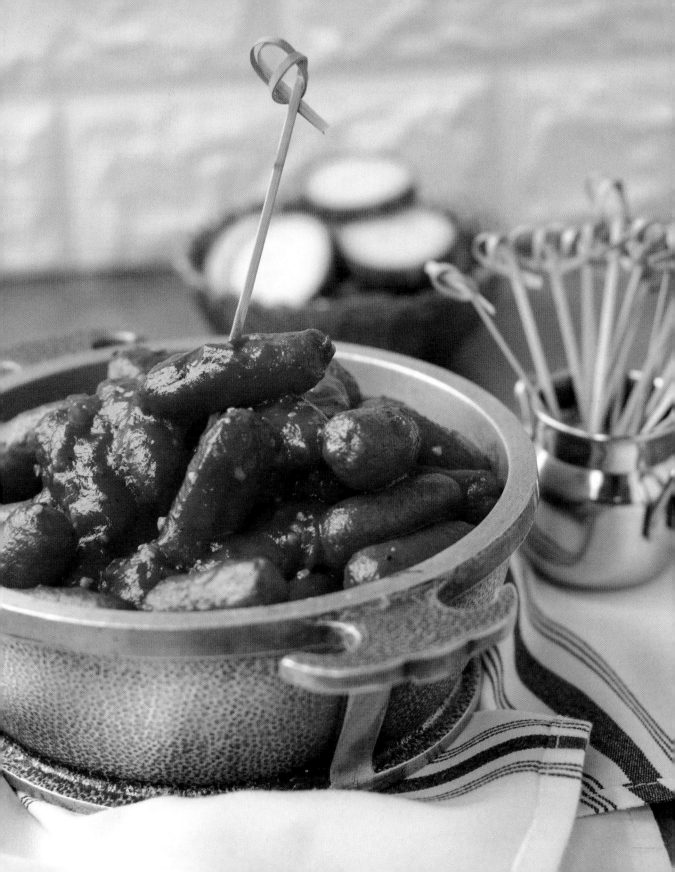

Bloody Mary Roasted Nuts

All the flavors of your favorite Sunday morning hangover cocktail, but in a deliciously crunchy snack.

Makes 3¼ cups (½ cup per serving) | Prep time: 10 minutes | Cook time: 20 minutes _____

¼ cup unsalted butter or ghee, melted

1 tablespoon tomato paste

1 tablespoon Worcestershire sauce

2 teaspoons hot sauce, such as Tapatío or Cholula

1 teaspoon garlic powder

1 teaspoon onion powder

½ teaspoon celery salt

3 cups roasted, salted mixed nuts

1 Preheat the oven to 350°F. Line a rimmed baking sheet with parchment paper or a silicone baking mat.

2 In a large mixing bowl, combine the butter, tomato paste, Worcestershire sauce, hot sauce, garlic powder, onion powder, and celery salt. Whisk to combine.

3 Add the nuts to the bowl and toss to coat. Mix until the nuts are evenly coated with the sauce.

4 Spread the nuts in a single layer across the prepared baking sheet. Roast for 20 minutes. Let cool before serving.

5 Store leftovers in an airtight container at room temperature for up to 2 weeks.

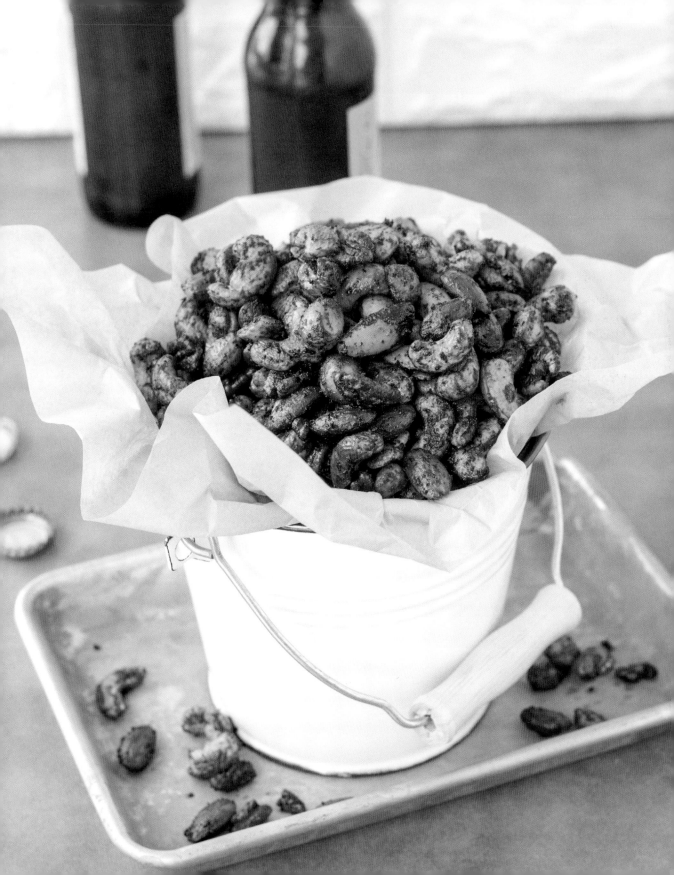

NET CARBS
3.6g

Buffalo Chicken Jalapeño Poppers

Two traditional bar snacks get a major makeover in this recipe. Instead of having to choose jalapeño poppers or Buffalo wings, how about getting both in one dish? Serve with some creamy ranch dressing on the side, and you've got a match made in heaven.

Makes 20 poppers (4 per serving) | Prep time: 15 minutes | Cook time: 35 minutes _____

10 large jalapeño peppers, halved lengthwise and seeded

8 ounces ground chicken

2 cloves garlic, minced

½ teaspoon onion powder

½ teaspoon fine sea salt

4 ounces full-fat cream cheese (½ cup), softened

½ cup crumbled blue cheese, divided

¼ cup shredded mozzarella cheese

¼ cup Buffalo wing sauce

4 slices bacon, cooked crisp and crumbled

2 green onions, sliced, for garnish

Ranch dressing, for serving

1 Preheat the oven to 350°F. Line a rimmed baking sheet with parchment paper or a silicone baking mat.

2 Spread the jalapeño halves across the lined baking sheet.

3 Heat a large skillet over medium heat. Add the ground chicken, garlic, onion powder, and salt and sauté until the chicken is cooked all the way through and is no longer pink.

4 Transfer the cooked chicken mixture to a large bowl. Add the cream cheese, ¼ cup of the blue cheese, the mozzarella, and the Buffalo wing sauce. Mix until the ingredients are well combined.

5 Fill each jalapeño half with a mound of the chicken mixture. Top with the remaining ¼ cup of blue cheese crumbles and the crumbled bacon.

6 Bake for 30 minutes, or until the tops are golden brown.

7 Garnish with the green onions and serve with ranch dressing.

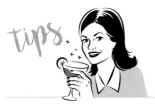

tips

If you can't find ground chicken at your local grocery store, feel free to substitute ground turkey.

For several different keto-friendly ranch dressing recipes, visit the dressings section of my website, peaceloveandlowcarb.com.

CALORIES: 252 | FAT: 19g | PROTEIN: 16g | TOTAL CARBS: 4.6g | DIETARY FIBER: 1g | NET CARBS: 3.6g

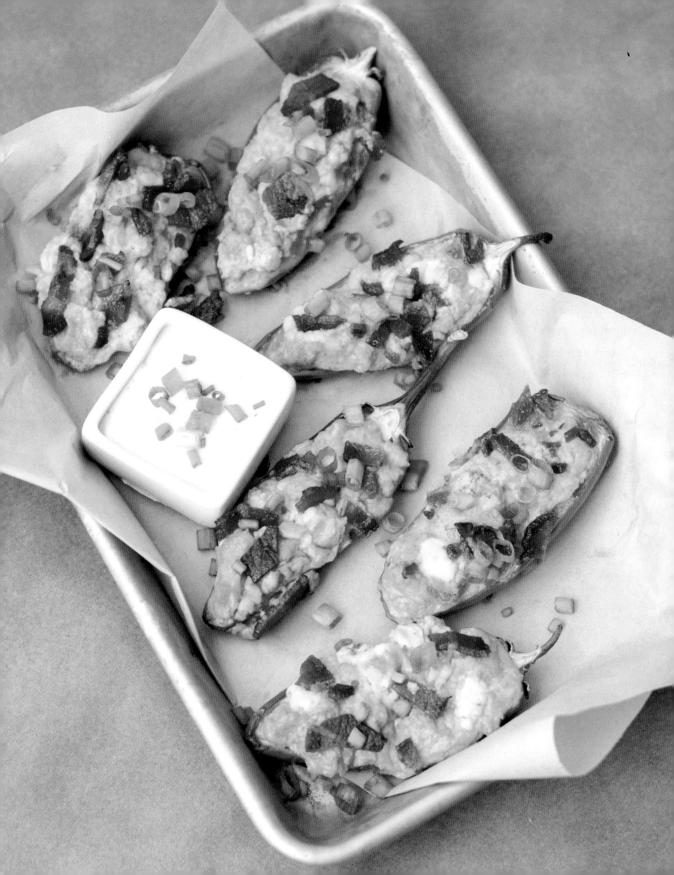

Cheesy Nachos

I bet you never thought you would be eating nachos again after switching to a low-carb ketogenic lifestyle. Well, I am happy to tell you that with a little creativity, anything is possible in the low-carb food world—even nachos. I love to kick back with a plate of these nachos and a Cucumber Jalapeño Margarita (page 100) on football Sundays.

Makes 4 servings | Prep time: 10 minutes, plus 40 minutes to cool | Cook time: 12 minutes ____

FOR THE CHIPS:

2 cups shredded sharp cheddar cheese

½ cup grated Parmesan cheese

1 teaspoon ground cumin

½ teaspoon garlic powder

¼ teaspoon chili powder

FOR THE NACHO PLATTER:

Chips (from above)

8 ounces ground beef, crumbled and cooked with taco seasoning (about 1 cup)

¼ cup shredded sharp cheddar cheese

¼ cup diced tomatoes

¼ cup sliced jalapeño peppers

¼ cup sliced black olives

¼ cup guacamole

¼ cup full-fat sour cream

2 tablespoons chopped onions

A few sprigs of fresh cilantro, for garnish (optional)

1 Place an oven rack in the middle of the oven. Preheat the oven to 400°F. Line a rimmed baking sheet with parchment paper or a silicone baking mat.

2 To make the chips, sprinkle the cheddar cheese on the parchment paper in a thin layer in a rectangle shape, about 13 by 9 inches. Sprinkle the Parmesan evenly over the cheddar cheese.

3 In a small bowl, combine the cumin, garlic powder, and chili powder. Sprinkle the seasoning mix evenly over the cheeses.

4 Bake for 8 to 10 minutes, until the cheese starts to brown ever so slightly, checking every minute to ensure that it does not burn. Remove from the oven and let cool for 10 minutes.

5 Peel the cooked cheese away from the parchment paper and cut it lengthwise into 2-inch-wide strips. A pizza cutter or kitchen shears makes this task easier. After cutting the cheese into strips, cut each strip into triangles.

6 Transfer the chips back to the parchment paper and broil on high for 1 to 2 minutes, until they start to bubble slightly and get crisp.

7 Remove the sheet of parchment paper with the chips on it from the baking sheet. Let the chips cool and crisp up, about 30 minutes.

8   To assemble the nacho platter, pile the chips on a plate and cover with the seasoned and cooked beef, cheese, tomatoes, jalapeños, olives, guacamole, sour cream, and onions. Garnish with cilantro, if using.

Crispy Baked
Garlic-Parmesan Wings

It is really hard to find a good crispy baked chicken wing recipe. Most of the recipes I have tried over the years ended up being a soft, chewy mess. The key to perfectly crispy wings lies in the technique. It's all about salting them first to draw out excess moisture from the skin, then coating them in baking powder, and then cooking them at two different temperatures on two different racks in the oven. The result is a golden and crispy outside and a juicy and tender inside. Once you make wings this way, you will never want to make them another way again. I love to serve these with ranch dressing. Delicious!

Makes 6 servings
Prep time: 10 minutes, plus 20 minutes to rest | Cook time: 1 hour 15 minutes _____

2 pounds chicken wings, thawed if frozen

1 teaspoon fine sea salt

2 tablespoons baking powder

FOR THE SAUCE:

½ cup salted butter, melted

½ cup grated Parmesan cheese

1 clove garlic, minced

1 tablespoon chopped fresh flat-leaf parsley

1½ teaspoons garlic powder

½ teaspoon onion powder

¼ teaspoon ground black pepper

1 Spread the wings in a single layer across some paper towels and sprinkle with the salt. Cover with another layer of paper towels and let rest for 20 minutes.

2 Place an oven rack in the middle-lower position and another rack in the middle-upper position. Preheat the oven to 250°F. Set a cooling rack on a rimmed baking sheet.

3 Combine the wings and baking powder in a resealable plastic bag. Shake to coat the wings evenly.

4 Spread the wings in a single layer across the cooling rack. Bake on the middle-lower oven rack for 30 minutes.

5 Increase the oven temperature to 425°F and move the baking sheet to the middle-upper rack. Bake the wings for an additional 45 minutes, or until the skin is nice and crispy.

6 While the wings are baking, make the sauce: Combine the melted butter, Parmesan cheese, minced garlic, parsley, garlic powder, onion powder, and pepper in a medium bowl.

7 Remove the wings from the oven and let rest for 5 minutes. Toss in the sauce before serving.

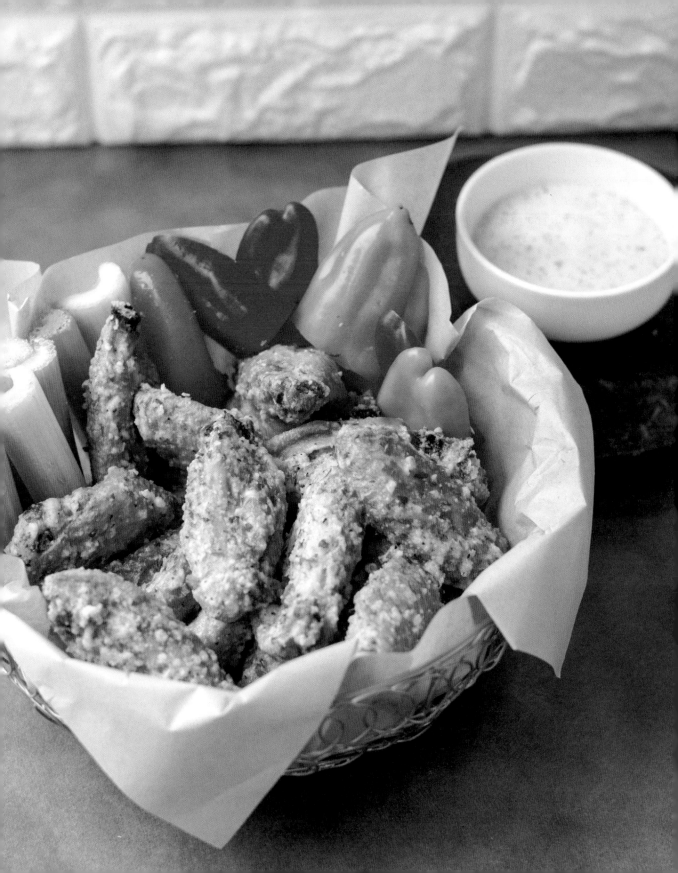

EATS AND
TREATS

 NET CARBS
2.7g

Grilled Halloumi Bruschetta

I am truly amazed by halloumi. It holds up to high heat and maintains its salty, meaty texture. And yet it is cheese. While it is amazing all on its own, it makes a truly great low-carb substitute for bread.

Makes 8 servings | Prep time: 20 minutes | Cook time: 5 minutes _____

FOR THE TOPPING:

1 medium tomato, diced

2 cloves garlic, minced

¼ cup chopped Kalamata olives

3 tablespoons grated Parmesan cheese

2 tablespoons capers

2 tablespoons chopped fresh basil, plus more for garnish

1 tablespoon avocado oil or olive oil

1 tablespoon balsamic vinegar

¼ teaspoon ground black pepper

FOR THE BASE:

8 ounces halloumi cheese

Avocado oil or olive oil, for the pan

1 Make the topping: In a large mixing bowl, combine the ingredients for the topping. Toss to combine. Set aside.

2 Cut the halloumi into 8 even slices.

3 Brush a grill pan with oil and heat over medium heat. When the pan is hot, lay the halloumi slices in a single layer across the pan.

4 Sear on both sides to create golden-brown grill marks and heat the cheese, about 2 minutes on each side.

5 Transfer the halloumi to a serving tray. Top each slice with the topping mixture and garnish with basil.

6 Store any leftovers in an airtight container in the refrigerator for up to 1 week.

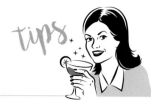

tips

If you don't have a grill pan, no problem! Simply pan-fry the halloumi slices until they are golden brown on both sides.

Leftover bruschetta are great eaten straight out of the fridge, but you can warm them if you prefer.

186 CALORIES: 170 | FAT: 14g | PROTEIN: 8.6g | TOTAL CARBS: 3g | DIETARY FIBER: 0.3g | NET CARBS: 2.7g

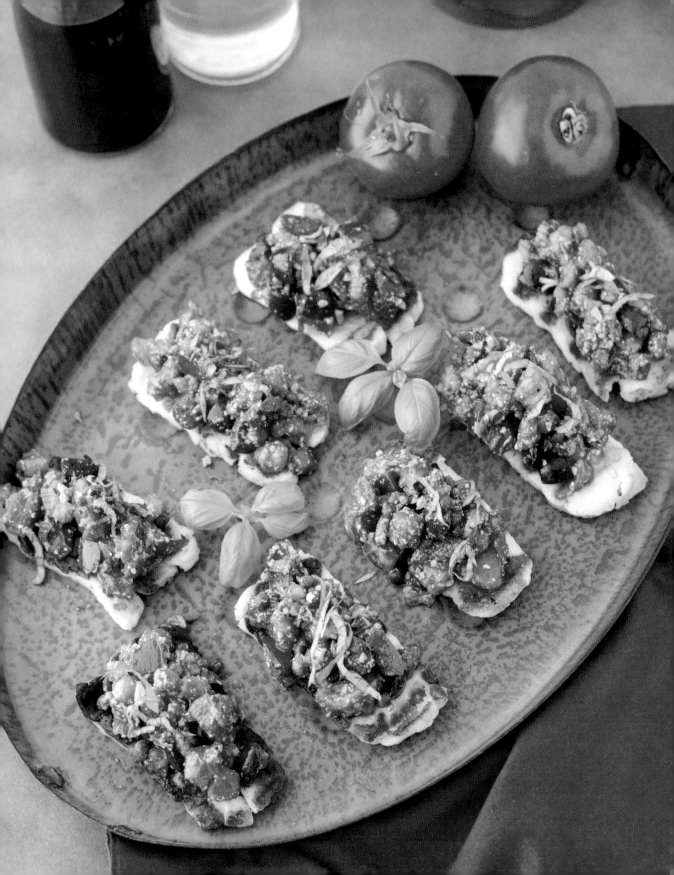

Keto Soft Pretzels

Soft pretzels remind me of walking into the mall as a teenager and passing the pretzel stand in the food court. It was like the aroma followed me all through the mall, calling to me. Well, now I can have my low-carb and gluten-free soft pretzel and eat it, too! I love to dip these pretzels in spicy brown mustard.

Makes 6 pretzels (1 per serving) | Prep time: 10 minutes | Cook time: 18 minutes _____

2 cups blanched almond flour

1 tablespoon baking powder

1 teaspoon garlic powder

1 teaspoon onion powder

3 large eggs, divided

3 cups shredded low-moisture, part-skim mozzarella cheese

2½ ounces full-fat cream cheese (5 tablespoons), softened

Coarse sea salt, for topping

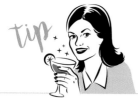

I love to enjoy these pretzels freshly baked and hot, but they are also amazing cold.

1 Preheat the oven to 425°F. Line a rimmed baking sheet with parchment paper or a silicone baking mat.

2 In a medium mixing bowl, whisk together the almond flour, baking powder, garlic powder, and onion powder until well combined.

3 Crack one of the eggs into a small bowl and whisk with a fork; set aside. (This will be the egg wash for the tops of the pretzels. The other 2 eggs will go into the dough.)

4 In a microwave-safe mixing bowl, combine the mozzarella and cream cheese. Microwave for 1 minute 30 seconds. Remove the bowl from the microwave and stir to combine. Return the bowl to the microwave for 1 more minute.

5 To the bowl with the cheeses, add the remaining 2 eggs and the almond flour mixture. Working the dough by hand, mix until the ingredients are well incorporated. If the dough gets too stringy and becomes unworkable, simply put it back in the microwave for 30 seconds to soften, then continue mixing. If the dough starts sticking to your hands, wet your hands just slightly and continue working the dough.

6 Divide the dough into 6 equal portions. Roll each portion into a long, thin rope that resembles a breadstick. Fold each one into the shape of a pretzel.

7 Brush the tops of the pretzels with the egg wash. Sprinkle coarse sea salt over the pretzels.

8 Bake for 12 to 14 minutes, until golden brown.

9 Store any leftovers in the refrigerator for up to 1 week. To reheat, place in a preheated 250°F oven until warmed through.

Pizza Bagels

I am a firm believer that even bad pizza is good pizza. Yes, I said it. You see, I just really, really love pizza. It was not something that I was willing to give up when I switched to a low-carb lifestyle. So what did I do? I created about twenty different variations of low-carb pizza, along with a terrific low-carb pizza sauce (which you can use on these bagels as well). All the recipes are on my website, peaceloveandlowcarb.com.

Makes 6 bagels (1 per serving) | Prep time: 15 minutes | Cook time: 15 minutes _____

2 cups blanched almond flour

1 tablespoon baking powder

1 teaspoon garlic powder

1 teaspoon onion powder

1 teaspoon Italian seasoning

3 cups shredded low-moisture, part-skim mozzarella cheese

1½ ounces full-fat cream cheese (3 tablespoons), softened

2 large eggs, whisked

2½ ounces pepperoni slices, chopped

¼ cup low-carb pizza sauce (see note), plus more for serving (optional)

1 teaspoon dried oregano leaves

2 tablespoons shredded Parmesan cheese

note

You can use store-bought pizza sauce or marinara sauce if you like. Just be sure to purchase a brand that is free of additives and added sugars. The only ingredients should be tomatoes, herbs, and spices. Or use the low-carb pizza sauce recipe on peaceloveandlowcarb.com for a delicious homemade version.

1   Preheat the oven to 425°F. Line a rimmed baking sheet with parchment paper or a silicone baking mat.

2   In a medium mixing bowl, whisk together the almond flour, baking powder, garlic powder, onion powder, and Italian seasoning until the ingredients are well combined.

3   In a large microwave-safe mixing bowl, combine the mozzarella and cream cheese. Microwave for 1 minute 30 seconds. Remove from the microwave and stir to combine. If the dough gets too stringy and becomes unworkable, simply put it back in the microwave for 30 seconds to soften, then continue mixing.

4   To the bowl with the cheeses, add the eggs and almond flour mixture. Working the dough by hand, mix until the ingredients are well incorporated. If you are having a hard time mixing the ingredients together, put the bowl back in the microwave for another 20 to 30 seconds to soften. If the dough starts sticking to your hands, wet your hands slightly and continue working the dough.

5   Once the dough is well combined, add the pepperoni and mix it in. Little by little, mix in the pizza sauce. The dough will be fairly soft.

6   Divide the dough into 6 equal portions. Using your hands, roll each portion into a ball.

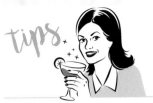

7　Gently press your finger through the center of each dough ball to form a ring. Stretch the ring to make a small hole (about 1 inch) in the center and form the dough into a bagel shape.

8　Top the bagels with the oregano and Parmesan cheese. Bake for 12 to 14 minutes, until golden brown. Serve with pizza sauce on the side, if desired.

9　Store any leftovers in an airtight container in the refrigerator for up to 1 week. To reheat, place in a preheated 250°F oven until warmed through.

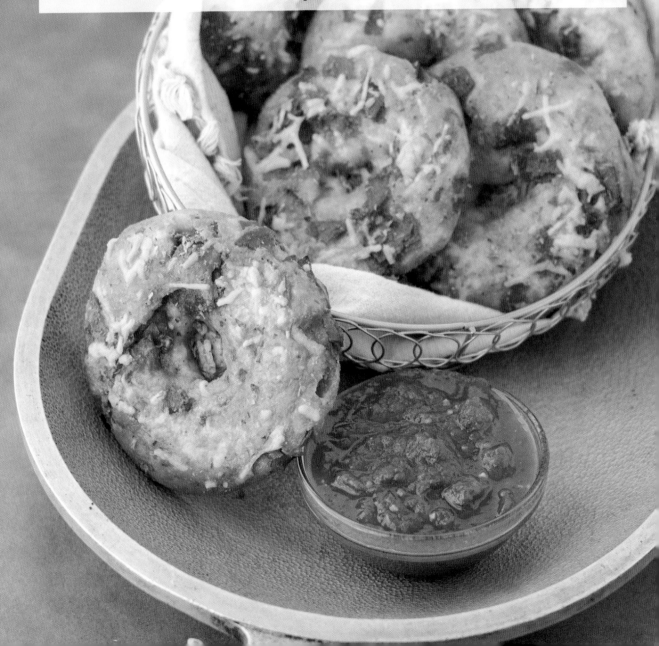

Pork Belly BLTC Stacks

Adding crispy pork belly is the perfect way to elevate a traditional BLT—it is smoky, salty, fatty deliciousness, just oozing with flavor and texture. Bring these stacks to your next potluck-style party; it is sure to be the first plate emptied.

Makes 12 stacks (2 per serving) | Prep time: 15 minutes | Cook time: 10 minutes _____

12 ounces fully cooked pork belly, cut into 12 large chunks

4 ounces sharp cheddar cheese, cut into 12 cubes

12 grape tomatoes

2 large romaine lettuce leaves, each torn into 6 pieces

Mayonnaise, for serving (optional)

SPECIAL EQUIPMENT:

12 (6-inch) bamboo cocktail skewers

1 Heat a cast-iron skillet over medium-high heat. Place the pork belly in the pan and cook until seared and crispy on all sides, about 10 minutes.

2 Remove the pork belly from the skillet and let it rest on a paper towel to absorb any excess grease.

3 Divide all the ingredients evenly among the 12 skewers, threading each skewer with a cheese cube, then a tomato, then a piece of lettuce, and finally a piece of pork belly.

4 Serve with mayonnaise for dipping, if desired.

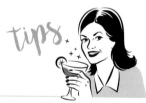

If using uncooked, unseasoned pork belly, season it generously with salt before cooking and pan-fry it until it is cooked through and the skin is nice and crispy.

Trader Joe's sells amazing precooked pork belly. It comes vacuum-sealed in 12-ounce packages and is perfect for recipes like this.

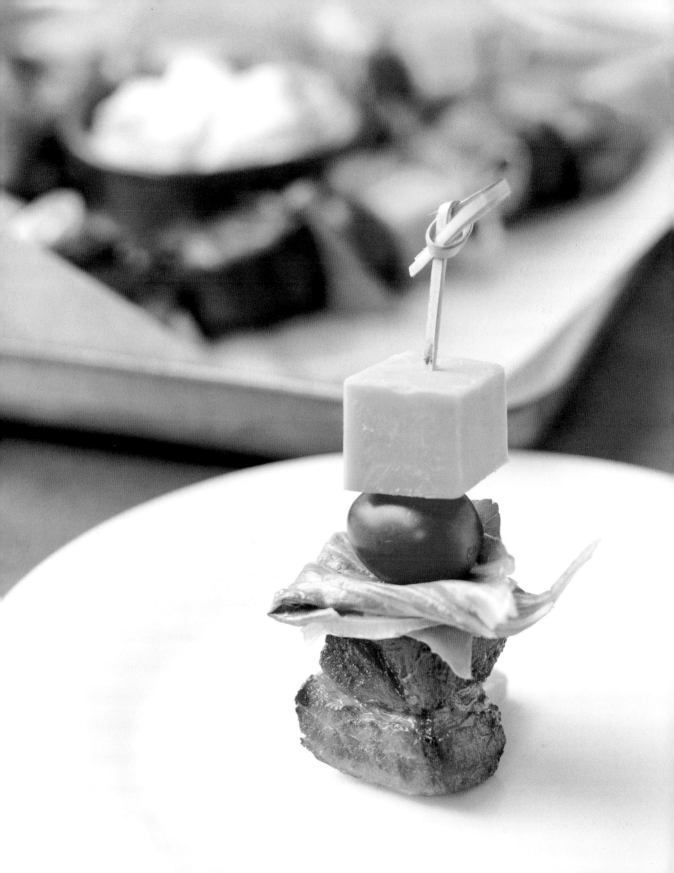

Teriyaki Steak Bites

These tender and juicy steak bites are the perfect amount of sweet, with just a hint of savory thrown into the mix. They make a great party appetizer, or add some steamed broccoli and cauliflower rice for a complete meal.

Makes 4 servings | Prep time: 10 minutes | Cook time: 20 minutes

1 pound boneless beef steak of choice, cut into large chunks

Fine sea salt and ground black pepper

2 tablespoons avocado oil or olive oil, for the pan

FOR THE SAUCE:

½ cup water, divided

¼ cup coconut aminos or gluten-free soy sauce

1 tablespoon unseasoned rice vinegar

2 tablespoons powdered erythritol

2 teaspoons brown sugar erythritol (optional)

2 cloves garlic, minced

1 teaspoon grated fresh ginger

½ teaspoon avocado oil or olive oil

1 teaspoon xanthan gum

5 large Bibb lettuce leaves, for lining the bowl (optional)

1 tablespoon toasted sesame seeds, for garnish

1 green onion, sliced on the bias, for garnish

1 Season the steak generously with salt and pepper.

2 Heat a large skillet over medium-high heat. Once hot, add the 2 tablespoons of oil. When the oil is hot, add the beef to the pan and sear on all sides. Remove the skillet from the heat and set aside.

3 Make the sauce: In a saucepan over medium-high heat, whisk together ¼ cup of the water, the coconut aminos, rice vinegar, powdered erythritol, brown sugar erythritol (if using), garlic, and ginger.

4 While the mixture is heating up, make the slurry: In a pint-sized glass, mix the remaining ¼ cup of water, the ½ teaspoon of oil, and the xanthan gum. Whisk vigorously to combine.

5 Pour the slurry into the sauce. Whisk continuously until you can no longer see any of the xanthan gum and the sauce starts to thicken. Reduce the heat to low and, stirring occasionally, simmer for 7 to 8 minutes, until the sauce is nice and thick.

6 Pour the sauce into the skillet with the steak and toss to coat. If you prefer your meat cooked beyond medium-rare, cook on medium-low until the steak has reached the desired level of doneness.

7 Line a large serving bowl with the lettuce leaves, if using, and top with the teriyaki steak. Garnish with the sesame seeds and green onions before serving.

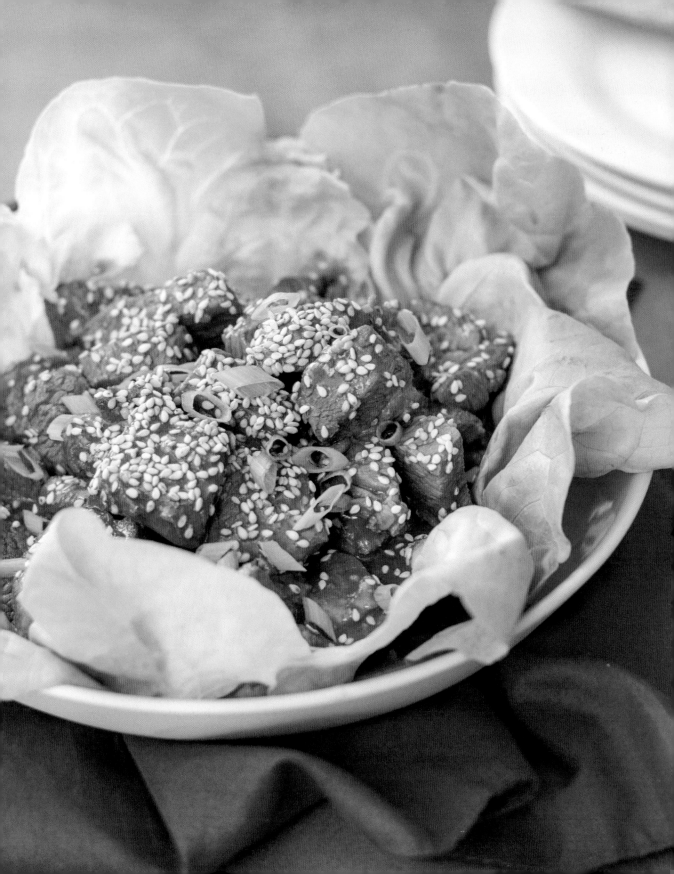

Red Wine Fudge Pops

A glass of bold red wine paired with a gluten-free fudgy, chocolaty dessert is one of my favorite flavor combinations in the world. I figured, why not combine them into an adult version of a childhood favorite?

Makes 10 fudge pops (1 per serving)
Prep time: 5 minutes, plus overnight to freeze | Cook time: 10 minutes _____

12 ounces dry red wine

½ cup sugar-free dark chocolate chips

4 ounces full-fat cream cheese (½ cup), softened

¾ cup heavy cream

⅓ cup powdered erythritol

2 tablespoons unsweetened cocoa powder

SPECIAL EQUIPMENT:
10 (3-ounce) ice pop molds

1 Bring the wine to a boil in a medium saucepan. Reduce the heat to low and simmer for 5 minutes.

2 Add the chocolate chips and cream cheese and whisk until fully melted and smooth.

3 Whisking continuously, add the cream, erythritol, and cocoa powder. Continue to whisk until the ingredients are well incorporated.

4 Transfer the mixture to a large liquid measuring cup with a pour spout. Divide it evenly among the ice pop molds.

5 Place a stick in each mold and freeze overnight.

6 Store the fudge pops in the freezer for up to 2 weeks.

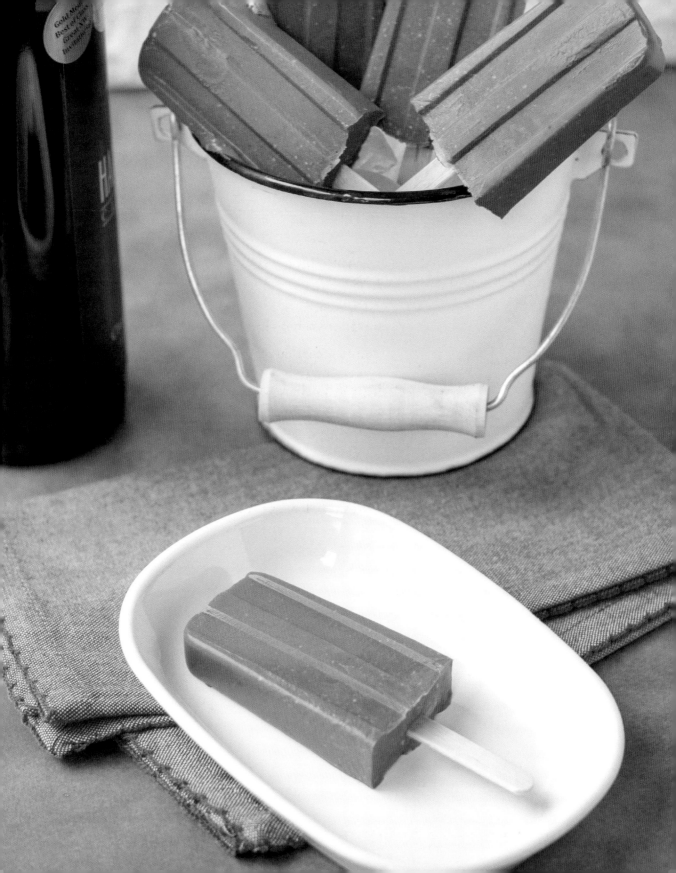

Recipe Index

MIXERS AND OTHER FUN STUFF

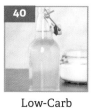

VODKA DRINKS

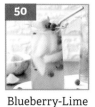
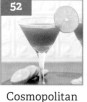

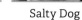
RUM DRINKS

GIN DRINKS

84
Blackberry-Basil Gin Fizz

86
Dirty Gibson

87
Gin Rickey

88
Grapefruit Dreamin'

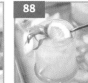
90
Lavender Ginny

92
Lemon-Basil Crush

94
Tom Collins

TEQUILA DRINKS

98
Bloody Maria

100
Cucumber-Jalapeño Margarita

102
Mama's Margarita

104
Pretty-in-Pink Paloma

106
Rosemary-Lime Tequila Spritzer

107
Brave Bull

108
Strawberry Margarita Gummy Worms

WHISKEY DRINKS

112 Irish Cold Brew

113 Whiskey Sour

114 It's Whiskey Thyme

116 Manhattan

118 Mint Julep

120 Old-Fashioned

122 Pickleback

123 Rosemary's Baby

WINE DRINKS

126 Lady in Red

128 Make It a Mimosa

130 Mixed Berry Prosecco Slushie

132 Raspberry-Mint Sparkler

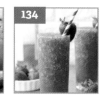
134 Strawberry Frosé

136 White Wine Spritzer

MIXIN' IT UP

140 Espresso Martini

142 French 75

144 Long Beach Iced Tea

145 Whiskey Sunset

146 Landslide

147 Black Russian

148 White Russian

149 Winearita

HOT DRINKS AND CORDIALS

152
Boosted and
Spiked Pumpkin
Spice Latte

154
Boozy
Hot Cocoa

156
Coffee-Spiked
Coffee

157
Hot Toddy

158
Flameless
Mexican Coffee

160
Hot Buttered
Rum

162
Irish Coffee

164
Homemade
Irish Cream
Liqueur

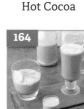
166
Homemade
Coffee Liqueur

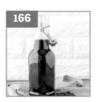

EATS AND TREATS

170
Antipasto Salad

172
Avocado
Hummus

174
Bacon and
Blue Cheese
Deviled Eggs

176
Barbecue
Cocktail
Sausages

178
Bloody Mary
Roasted Nuts

180
Buffalo Chicken
Jalapeño
Poppers

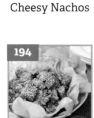
182
Cheesy Nachos

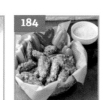
184
Crispy Baked
Garlic-Parmesan
Wings

186
Grilled
Halloumi
Bruschetta

188
Keto
Soft Pretzels

190
Pizza Bagels

192
Pork Belly
BLTC Stacks

194
Teriyaki
Steak Bites

196
Red Wine
Fudge Pops

General Index

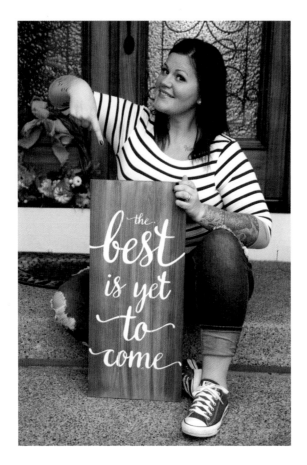

Kyndra Holley is the face behind the keyboard at *Peace, Love and Low Carb.* What started as a hobby blog and personal weight-loss journal now gets nearly 2 million page views per month. Kyndra's focus is on easy-to-make low-carb and gluten-free comfort food, and through her recipes and candid stories of her own struggles with weight, she has helped thousands of people lose weight and live healthier lives. Her previous publications include *Craveable Keto Cookbook, The Primal Low Carb Kitchen Cookbook,* and several other self-published works, as well as low-carb and gluten-free meal plans.

Kyndra's mission is to show people that a low-carb lifestyle is anything but restrictive and boring. When she is not in the kitchen working her food magic, she can often be found traveling the world with her partner in crime and husband, Jon, lifting weights, doing yoga, or playing with her five crazy pups. Kyndra resides in the beautiful Pacific Northwest, just outside of Seattle, Washington. For more of her recipes, visit peaceloveandlowcarb.com.